Castor Oil

For

Hair Growth

Bible

Ultimate Guide to

Thicker, Stronger, and Healthier Hair Naturally

Lucy Collins

Disclaimer

The information provided in this book is for informational purposes only. The content is not intended to be a substitute for professional medical advice, diagnosis, or treatment. Always seek the advice of your physician or other qualified health providers with any questions you may have regarding a medical condition or treatment. Never disregard professional medical advice or delay in seeking it because of something you have read in this book.

The author and publisher of this book disclaim any liability for any adverse effects, injuries, or damages arising directly or indirectly from the use or application of any information contained herein. The use of any information provided in this book is solely at your own risk.

This book does not provide medical or professional advice and should not be relied upon for such purposes. Readers are urged to consult with their healthcare provider or a qualified professional before making any decisions related to their health or treatment. The author and publisher do not accept any responsibility or liability for the accuracy, completeness, or usefulness of the information contained in this book.

Table of content

Introduction

Welcome to the Castor Oil for Hair Growth Bible

Welcome to the "Castor Oil for Hair Growth Bible." This comprehensive guide is designed to be your ultimate resource for achieving thicker, stronger, and healthier hair naturally. In a world saturated with synthetic products and quick-fix solutions, it is refreshing to return to the roots of hair care—embracing the power of nature and the time-tested benefits of castor oil.

Hair care is an essential aspect of personal grooming and overall well-being. Our hair not only enhances our physical appearance but also reflects our inner health and vitality. Therefore, taking care of our hair is not just about vanity; it is about nurturing a part of ourselves that speaks volumes about who we are.

The significance of hair care extends far beyond aesthetic appeal. Healthy hair can boost self-confidence, positively impacting our personal and professional lives. Conversely, hair problems such as thinning, breakage, and scalp issues can lead to a decline in self-esteem and even affect our emotional health. Understanding the importance of hair care is the first step towards achieving beautiful, resilient hair.

Hair care is a journey that involves understanding the unique needs of your hair and providing it with the right nutrients and treatments. In this book, you will find scientifically-backed information and practical advice on how to care for your hair using natural ingredients, with a special focus on castor oil. Castor oil, known for its remarkable properties, has been used for centuries to promote hair growth and improve hair health. This book will delve into the science behind castor oil, its benefits, and practical applications, providing you with all the knowledge you need to incorporate this powerful natural remedy into your hair care routine.

Healthy hair is a reflection of overall well-being. It signifies that the body is well-nourished, free from stress, and balanced. By focusing on holistic hair care practices, you are not only enhancing your appearance but also fostering a healthier lifestyle. Proper hair care routines can prevent common issues like hair loss, dandruff, and dullness, leading to long-lasting results.

In the following pages, you will discover the secrets of castor oil, understand its profound impact on hair health, and learn how to use it effectively. Whether you are dealing with hair loss, thinning hair, or simply seeking to enhance your hair's strength and shine, this book offers solutions that are both natural and effective.

Join us on this journey to uncover the benefits of castor oil for hair growth. Let's explore the science, debunk the myths, and embrace the natural path to beautiful, healthy hair.

Overview of the benefits of castor oil

Castor oil, derived from the seeds of the Ricinus communis plant, is a natural elixir with a rich history of use in traditional medicine and beauty practices. Its numerous benefits make it an essential ingredient in many hair care regimens. This section provides a comprehensive overview of the remarkable advantages of incorporating castor oil into your hair care routine.

1. Promotes Hair Growth

One of the most celebrated benefits of castor oil is its ability to promote hair growth. Rich in ricinoleic acid, a type of fatty acid that acts as a potent anti-inflammatory agent, castor oil helps improve blood circulation to the scalp. Enhanced circulation ensures that hair follicles receive the necessary nutrients and oxygen, which can stimulate hair growth. Regular application of castor oil can result in visibly thicker and longer hair over time.

2. Strengthens Hair

Castor oil is known for its deep conditioning properties, which can significantly strengthen the hair shaft. The high concentration of omega-6 and omega-9 fatty acids, along with vitamin E, penetrates the hair cuticle to provide intense nourishment. This helps to fortify the hair strands, reducing breakage and split ends. Stronger hair is less prone to damage, making it look healthier and more resilient.

3. Moisturizes and Conditions

Dry and brittle hair is a common problem that can lead to further hair issues. Castor oil is an excellent natural moisturizer due to its high viscosity and emollient properties. It forms a protective barrier on the hair and scalp, locking in moisture and preventing dehydration. As a result, hair feels softer, more manageable, and has a natural shine. The conditioning effects of castor oil also help to smooth frizz and improve the overall texture of the hair.

4. Treats Scalp Conditions

A healthy scalp is the foundation of healthy hair. Castor oil has antimicrobial and antifungal properties that can address various scalp conditions such as dandruff, scalp infections, and seborrheic dermatitis. The anti-inflammatory properties of ricinoleic acid help soothe irritated scalp skin, reducing itching and flaking. By maintaining a clean and balanced scalp environment, castor oil promotes the growth of strong and healthy hair.

5. Enhances Hair Flexibility and Elasticity

Hair flexibility and elasticity are crucial for preventing breakage during styling and manipulation. The fatty acids in castor oil penetrate the hair shaft, increasing its elasticity and flexibility. This makes the hair more resistant to physical stress and reduces the likelihood of damage from brushing, combing, and styling tools. Enhanced elasticity also contributes to the overall strength and health of the hair.

6. Provides Antioxidant Protection

Castor oil is rich in antioxidants, particularly vitamin E, which plays a vital role in protecting the hair from environmental damage. Antioxidants neutralize free radicals that can cause oxidative stress, leading to hair damage and premature aging. By protecting the hair from such damage, castor oil helps maintain its youthful appearance and vitality.

7. Supports Hair Regeneration

For those experiencing hair loss or thinning, castor oil can support hair regeneration. Its nutrient-rich composition nourishes the hair follicles, potentially reactivating dormant follicles and promoting the growth of new hair. Regular use of castor oil can help in the recovery of lost hair density and volume, making it an effective remedy for thinning hair.

Incorporating castor oil into your hair care routine can yield significant improvements in hair health and appearance. Whether used alone or in combination with other natural ingredients, castor oil offers a holistic approach to hair care, addressing various issues from the root to the tip.

Purpose of the Book

Explanation of the book's aim

The purpose of the "Castor Oil for Hair Growth Bible" is to provide an all-encompassing guide to understanding and utilizing the potent benefits of castor oil for hair health. This book aims to demystify the science behind castor oil, offering readers clear, evidence-based information and practical advice on how to incorporate this natural remedy into their hair care routines. By bridging the gap between traditional wisdom and modern science, this book seeks to empower readers to make informed decisions about their hair care practices.

Empowering Informed Decisions

Many individuals struggle with various hair problems, ranging from hair loss and thinning to scalp conditions and lackluster hair. The beauty industry is flooded with products promising miraculous results, often at the cost of exposing hair to harsh chemicals and synthetic ingredients. This book advocates for a return to natural solutions, specifically highlighting the unmatched benefits of castor oil. By understanding the properties and applications of castor oil, readers can make informed choices that align with their health and beauty goals.

Comprehensive Knowledge Resource

This book serves as a comprehensive resource for anyone looking to improve their hair health. It covers a wide range of topics, including the science of hair growth, the structure and function of hair, and the various factors that affect hair health. Readers will gain a deep understanding of how castor oil works, its chemical composition, and the historical context of its use. The aim is to equip readers with a solid foundation of knowledge, enabling them to use castor oil effectively and confidently.

Practical Applications and Techniques

Beyond the theoretical knowledge, this book is packed with practical advice and step-by-step instructions. Readers will learn how to select the right type of castor oil, prepare it for use, and apply it using various techniques. Detailed guidelines on frequency and dosage ensure that users can maximize the benefits without overuse. Additionally, the book offers a variety of DIY recipes for hair masks, conditioners, and serums, allowing readers to customize their hair care regimen according to their specific needs.

Holistic Approach to Hair Health

Understanding that hair health is not solely dependent on topical treatments, this book adopts a holistic approach. It explores the importance of a healthy lifestyle, including diet, nutrition, and stress management, in promoting optimal hair growth. By integrating these lifestyle practices with castor oil treatments, readers can achieve sustainable and long-lasting improvements in their hair health.

Success Stories and Real-Life Testimonials

To inspire and motivate readers, the book includes real-life success stories and testimonials from individuals who have experienced the transformative effects of castor oil. These personal accounts provide valuable insights and reinforce the effectiveness of the methods discussed. Before-and-after case studies offer concrete examples of the positive outcomes that can be achieved with regular use of castor oil.

A Trusted Companion in Your Hair Care Journey

Ultimately, the goal of this book is to be a trusted companion in your hair care journey. Whether you are new to the world of natural hair care or a seasoned enthusiast, the "Castor Oil for Hair Growth Bible" aims to support you every step of the way. By providing reliable information, practical tips, and motivational stories, this book encourages readers to embrace the natural path to beautiful, healthy hair.

We hope that this book not only enhances your understanding of castor oil but also inspires you to explore the broader world of natural hair care. Together, we can rediscover the beauty and effectiveness of nature's gifts, leading to a healthier, more radiant you.

What the readers can expect to gain

The "Castor Oil for Hair Growth Bible" is designed to be an invaluable resource for anyone seeking to improve their hair health through natural means. Here's what you can expect to gain from this comprehensive guide:

1. In-Depth Knowledge of Hair and Hair Growth

Understanding the fundamentals of hair biology is crucial for effective hair care. This book delves into the science of hair growth, explaining the structure and composition of hair, the hair growth cycle, and the various factors that influence hair health. You will gain a clear understanding of how hair grows, why it stops growing, and what you can do to maintain its health and vitality.

2. Insight into Common Hair Problems and Solutions

Hair loss, thinning, and damage are common concerns for many people. This book addresses these issues head-on, providing detailed explanations of the causes and offering practical solutions. You will learn about the different types of hair loss, the reasons behind thinning hair, and the best practices for repairing damaged hair. With this knowledge, you will be better equipped to tackle your specific hair challenges.

3. Comprehensive Overview of Natural Hair Care

Natural hair care is gaining popularity for its gentle and sustainable approach. This book highlights the benefits of natural hair care over synthetic alternatives. You will discover key natural ingredients that promote hair health, including herbs, oils, and other botanicals. The focus on castor oil will provide you with a deep appreciation of its unique properties and benefits, making it a cornerstone of your hair care regimen.

4. Detailed Understanding of Castor Oil

Castor oil is a powerful natural remedy with a rich history. This book covers everything you need to know about castor oil, from its origins and types to its chemical composition and benefits. You will learn how castor oil promotes hair growth, strengthens hair, moisturizes, and conditions, and treats scalp conditions. This comprehensive understanding will empower you to use castor oil effectively and confidently.

5. Practical Application Techniques

Knowing how to use castor oil is as important as knowing its benefits. This book provides step-by-step instructions on how to prepare and apply castor oil. You will learn various application techniques, including scalp massages, overnight treatments, and hot oil treatments. Detailed frequency and dosage recommendations ensure that you can use castor oil safely and effectively.

6. DIY Recipes and Hair Treatments

Customization is key to effective hair care. This book offers a range of DIY recipes for hair masks, conditioners, serums, and sprays. These recipes combine castor oil with other beneficial ingredients, allowing you to tailor treatments to your specific needs. You will also find tips on combining castor oil with essential oils, carrier oils, and herbal infusions to enhance its effects.

7. Holistic Approach to Hair Health

Healthy hair is a reflection of a healthy lifestyle. This book explores the role of diet, nutrition, and stress management in promoting hair growth. You will gain insights into how lifestyle factors influence hair health and learn practical strategies for integrating healthy practices into your daily routine. This holistic approach ensures that you are addressing hair health from the inside out.

8. Inspiration from Success Stories

Real-life success stories and testimonials provide inspiration and motivation. This book includes personal accounts from individuals who have experienced the transformative effects of castor oil. These stories, along with before-and-after case studies, offer concrete evidence of the positive outcomes that can be achieved. They serve as a reminder that natural hair care is not only effective but also accessible.

9. A Trusted Resource for Ongoing Hair Care

The "Castor Oil for Hair Growth Bible" is designed to be a trusted companion on your hair care journey. Whether you are a beginner or a seasoned natural hair care enthusiast, this book offers valuable information and guidance. It aims to support you in achieving your hair goals and maintaining healthy hair in the long term.

By the end of this book, you will have a thorough understanding of how to care for your hair naturally, using the powerful benefits of castor oil. You will be equipped with the knowledge, techniques, and inspiration to transform your hair health and embrace a natural approach to beauty.

Part I

Understanding Hair and Hair Growth

The Science of Hair Growth

Hair Structure and Composition

Detailed explanation of hair anatomy

To fully appreciate the benefits of castor oil for hair growth, it is essential to understand the intricate structure and composition of hair. Hair is a complex biological material composed of several layers and components, each playing a crucial role in its overall health and growth.

1. Hair Shaft

The hair shaft is the visible part of the hair that extends above the scalp. It is made up of three distinct layers:

- **Cuticle:** The outermost layer, the cuticle, is composed of overlapping, scale-like cells that protect the inner layers of the hair. A healthy cuticle is smooth and flat, reflecting light to give hair its natural shine. The cuticle also acts as a barrier against environmental damage and moisture loss.
- **Cortex:** Beneath the cuticle lies the cortex, which makes up the bulk of the hair shaft. The cortex contains tightly packed keratin fibers, providing strength, elasticity, and color to the hair. The pigment melanin, found in the cortex, determines hair color and can be affected by genetic factors and aging.
- **Medulla:** The innermost layer of the hair shaft, the medulla, is composed of a soft, spongy core. Not all hair types have a medulla, and its presence and function can vary among individuals. The medulla is more prominent in thicker, coarser hair.

2. Hair Follicle

The hair follicle is a tunnel-shaped structure embedded in the scalp that surrounds the root of the hair. It is responsible for hair growth and houses several key components:

- **Hair Bulb:** Located at the base of the follicle, the hair bulb is where hair growth begins. It contains living cells that divide and grow to form the hair shaft. The hair bulb is nourished by blood vessels that deliver essential nutrients and oxygen, supporting hair growth.
- **Dermal Papilla:** The dermal papilla is a cluster of specialized cells at the base of the hair bulb. These cells play a critical role in regulating hair growth by interacting with the surrounding follicle cells. They also help transfer nutrients from the bloodstream to the hair bulb.
- **Sebaceous Glands:** Attached to the hair follicle are sebaceous glands that secrete sebum, an oily substance that lubricates the hair and scalp. Sebum helps maintain moisture balance, preventing dryness and protecting the hair from environmental damage.

- **Arrector Pili Muscle:** This small, involuntary muscle is attached to the hair follicle. When it contracts, it causes the hair to stand upright, resulting in "goosebumps." This response is typically triggered by cold or emotional stimuli.

3. Hair Growth Cycle

Hair growth follows a cyclical pattern consisting of three main phases:

- **Anagen Phase (Growth Phase):** The anagen phase is the active growth phase of the hair cycle. During this period, hair cells in the bulb rapidly divide, pushing the hair shaft upward and out of the follicle. This phase can last anywhere from two to six years, depending on genetics and individual factors. Approximately 85-90% of hair follicles are in the anagen phase at any given time.
- **Catagen Phase (Transition Phase):** The catagen phase is a short transitional phase that lasts about two to three weeks. During this phase, hair growth slows down, and the hair follicle begins to shrink. The lower part of the hair follicle detaches from the dermal papilla, cutting off the blood supply to the hair bulb.
- **Telogen Phase (Resting Phase):** The telogen phase is the resting phase of the hair cycle, lasting about two to three months. During this period, the hair follicle remains inactive, and the hair shaft is fully formed. At the end of the telogen phase, the old hair is shed, and a new hair begins to grow, re-entering the anagen phase and starting the cycle anew.

4. Factors Affecting Hair Growth

Several factors can influence the hair growth cycle and the overall health of hair:

- **Genetics:** Genetic predisposition plays a significant role in determining hair growth patterns, hair thickness, and susceptibility to conditions such as androgenetic alopecia (pattern baldness).
- **Hormones:** Hormonal fluctuations, particularly androgens (male hormones), can impact hair growth. Conditions such as pregnancy, menopause, and thyroid disorders can also affect hair health.
- **Nutrition:** Adequate nutrition is essential for healthy hair growth. Nutrients such as vitamins (A, C, D, E), minerals (iron, zinc), and proteins (keratin) are vital for maintaining hair health and promoting growth.
- **Stress:** Chronic stress can disrupt the hair growth cycle, leading to conditions such as telogen effluvium, where a large number of hairs enter the telogen phase prematurely, resulting in noticeable hair shedding.
- **Medical Conditions:** Certain medical conditions, including autoimmune diseases, scalp infections, and chronic illnesses, can adversely affect hair growth.

Understanding the structure and composition of hair is the foundation for effective hair care. By appreciating the complexity of hair anatomy and the factors that influence its growth, you can make informed decisions to nurture and protect your hair.

Role of each component in hair health

To fully comprehend how to care for your hair effectively, it's essential to understand the role of each component within the hair structure. Each part of the hair and hair follicle contributes uniquely to hair health and its overall appearance. Here, we break down the role of each component in maintaining healthy hair.

1. Cuticle

The cuticle is the hair's outermost layer, consisting of overlapping, scale-like cells. Its primary roles include:

- **Protection:** The cuticle acts as a barrier that protects the inner layers of the hair from environmental damage such as UV radiation, pollution, and chemical exposure from hair treatments.
- **Moisture Retention:** A healthy cuticle layer helps retain moisture within the hair shaft, preventing dryness and brittleness. When the cuticle is smooth and intact, it reduces water loss and keeps the hair hydrated.
- **Strength and Shine:** The smoothness of the cuticle contributes to the hair's natural shine and strength. A well-maintained cuticle layer reflects light, giving hair its luster and smooth appearance.

2. Cortex

The cortex is the thickest layer of the hair shaft and is responsible for many of its key properties:

- **Strength and Elasticity:** The cortex contains long chains of keratin, a protein that gives hair its strength and elasticity. Healthy hair can stretch without breaking, thanks to the integrity of the keratin fibers.
- **Color:** The cortex houses melanin, the pigment responsible for hair color. The type and amount of melanin determine whether your hair is black, brown, blonde, or red. Melanin also provides some protection against UV damage.
- **Texture and Curl:** The shape and distribution of cells within the cortex influence hair texture, determining whether hair is straight, wavy, or curly. Variations in the cortex structure contribute to these differences.

3. Medulla

The medulla is the innermost layer of the hair shaft and is often absent in finer hair types. When present, its roles include:

- **Structural Integrity:** The medulla provides additional structural integrity to thick and coarse hair types. It acts as a core that supports the hair shaft.
- **Insulation:** The medulla can aid in insulating the hair, although its overall contribution to hair health is less significant compared to the cuticle and cortex.

4. Hair Follicle

The hair follicle is a complex structure beneath the scalp's surface and plays a critical role in hair growth and health:

- **Hair Bulb:** The hair bulb at the base of the follicle contains living cells that divide and grow to form the hair shaft. This area is where hair production begins, supported by nutrients supplied by the blood vessels.
- **Dermal Papilla:** Located within the hair bulb, the dermal papilla interacts with follicle cells to regulate hair growth. It supplies essential nutrients and growth factors that stimulate hair production.
- **Sebaceous Glands:** These glands produce sebum, an oily substance that conditions the scalp and hair. Sebum helps to maintain the scalp's moisture balance, preventing dryness and protecting the hair from becoming brittle.
- **Arrector Pili Muscle:** This small muscle is attached to the hair follicle. When it contracts, it causes the hair to stand upright, which can be a response to cold or emotional stimuli. While this muscle's role in hair health is minimal, it is part of the body's broader physiological responses.

5. Blood Supply and Nutrients

A healthy blood supply to the scalp is vital for hair health:

- **Nutrient Delivery:** Blood vessels surrounding the hair follicles deliver essential nutrients, including vitamins, minerals, and oxygen, which are crucial for hair growth and maintenance. Nutrient deficiencies can lead to weakened hair and slow growth.
- **Growth Stimulation:** Adequate blood flow ensures that hair follicles receive growth-promoting signals. Improved circulation can enhance the delivery of these signals, supporting robust hair growth.

6. Sebaceous Glands and Sebum Production

Sebaceous glands play a pivotal role in maintaining scalp and hair health:

- **Moisturization:** Sebum produced by these glands keeps both the scalp and hair shaft moisturized. It forms a protective layer that prevents excessive water loss and maintains the hair's flexibility.
- **Protection:** Sebum has antimicrobial properties that protect the scalp from infections. It also helps in keeping the scalp's pH balanced, creating an environment less conducive to harmful microbes.

7. Scalp Health

The health of the scalp is fundamental to the health of hair:

- **Cleanliness:** Regular cleansing of the scalp removes excess oil, dead skin cells, and product buildup that can clog hair follicles and inhibit growth.

- **pH Balance:** Maintaining the scalp's pH balance is essential for preventing issues such as dandruff and scalp irritation. A balanced pH supports a healthy environment for hair follicles to thrive.

Each component of the hair and hair follicle works in harmony to ensure the overall health and appearance of your hair. Understanding these roles can help you make more informed decisions about hair care practices and treatments, including the effective use of natural remedies like castor oil. By nurturing each part of the hair structure, you can promote stronger, healthier, and more resilient hair.

Hair Growth Cycle

Stages of hair growth

The hair growth cycle is a continuous process involving the growth, rest, and shedding of hair. Understanding this cycle is crucial for comprehending how to maintain healthy hair and effectively address hair growth issues. The hair growth cycle consists of three main stages: anagen, catagen, and telogen. Each stage has distinct characteristics and plays a vital role in the lifecycle of hair.

1. Anagen Phase (Growth Phase)

The anagen phase is the active growth phase of the hair cycle. During this period, hair cells in the bulb rapidly divide, pushing the hair shaft upward and out of the follicle. The anagen phase is characterized by:

- **Active Growth:** Hair grows approximately 1 centimeter per month during this phase. The duration of the anagen phase determines the maximum length of the hair.
- **Duration:** The anagen phase can last between two to six years, depending on genetics and individual factors. Some people may experience even longer growth phases, allowing their hair to grow much longer.
- **Percentage of Hair in Anagen:** At any given time, about 85-90% of hair follicles are in the anagen phase. This high percentage ensures continuous hair growth.

Role in Hair Health: The anagen phase is crucial for maintaining hair density and length. Factors such as genetics, nutrition, and overall health influence the length and quality of the anagen phase. A longer anagen phase results in longer hair, while a shorter phase can lead to shorter hair and potential thinning.

2. Catagen Phase (Transition Phase)

The catagen phase is a short, transitional phase that marks the end of active hair growth. During this period, the hair follicle undergoes significant changes:

- **Regression:** The hair follicle shrinks and detaches from the dermal papilla, cutting off the blood supply to the hair bulb. This process marks the end of active hair growth.
- **Duration:** The catagen phase lasts for about two to three weeks. It is a relatively brief phase compared to the anagen and telogen phases.
- **Percentage of Hair in Catagen:** Approximately 1-2% of hair follicles are in the catagen phase at any given time.

Role in Hair Health: The catagen phase allows the hair follicle to renew itself. This renewal is essential for the health of the hair follicle, ensuring it can produce new hair in subsequent cycles. Any disruptions to this phase can affect the overall health and productivity of the follicle.

3. Telogen Phase (Resting Phase)

The telogen phase is the resting phase of the hair cycle. During this period, the hair follicle remains inactive, and the hair shaft is fully formed:

- **Resting:** Hair does not grow during the telogen phase. The hair follicle is dormant, and the old hair remains in place until it is eventually shed.
- **Duration:** The telogen phase typically lasts about two to three months. This phase provides a period of rest for the hair follicle before it re-enters the anagen phase.
- **Percentage of Hair in Telogen:** About 10-15% of hair follicles are in the telogen phase at any given time.

Role in Hair Health: The telogen phase is essential for the natural shedding and renewal of hair. It ensures that old, damaged hair is replaced by new growth. An extended telogen phase can lead to increased shedding and noticeable thinning if new hair growth does not keep pace with shedding.

4. Exogen Phase (Shedding Phase)

Although not traditionally included as one of the primary stages, the exogen phase is considered by some experts as a separate phase where the hair is actively shed from the scalp:

- **Shedding:** During the exogen phase, hair that has reached the end of its telogen phase is shed from the scalp. This shedding allows new hair to emerge from the follicle.
- **Overlap with Telogen:** The exogen phase overlaps with the telogen phase, as new anagen hair begins to grow even before the old hair is shed.

Role in Hair Health: The exogen phase is a natural part of the hair renewal process. Shedding old hair allows new, healthy hair to take its place, maintaining the density and quality of the hair.

Factors Influencing the Hair Growth Cycle

Several factors can influence the duration and effectiveness of each phase in the hair growth cycle:

- **Genetics:** Genetic factors largely determine the length of the anagen phase and the overall hair growth cycle. Family history can predict hair growth patterns and susceptibility to hair loss conditions.
- **Hormones:** Hormonal changes, particularly androgens, can significantly impact the hair growth cycle. Conditions such as pregnancy, menopause, and thyroid disorders can alter the balance of hormones, affecting hair growth.
- **Nutrition:** Adequate nutrition is vital for healthy hair growth. Deficiencies in vitamins (such as A, C, D, and E), minerals (such as iron and zinc), and proteins can disrupt the hair growth cycle, leading to weakened hair and increased shedding.
- **Stress:** Chronic stress can lead to conditions such as telogen effluvium, where a large number of hairs enter the telogen phase prematurely, resulting in noticeable hair shedding.
- **Medical Conditions:** Certain medical conditions, including autoimmune diseases, scalp infections, and chronic illnesses, can adversely affect the hair growth cycle, leading to hair loss and thinning.

Factors influencing each stage

The hair growth cycle is dynamic and can be influenced by various internal and external factors. Understanding these influences can help you optimize hair growth and address issues related to hair health. Here we explore the key factors affecting each stage of the hair growth cycle.

1. Anagen Phase (Growth Phase)

The anagen phase is the period of active hair growth. Several factors can influence the duration and quality of this phase:

- **Genetics:** Genetic predisposition is a primary determinant of the length of the anagen phase. People with a family history of long hair growth cycles may experience longer anagen phases, allowing their hair to grow longer before transitioning to the next phase.
- **Hormonal Balance:** Hormones play a significant role in regulating the anagen phase. Androgens, particularly dihydrotestosterone (DHT), can shorten the anagen phase in individuals predisposed to androgenetic alopecia (pattern baldness). Conversely, higher levels of growth-promoting hormones can prolong the anagen phase.
- **Nutrition:** Adequate nutrition is crucial for maintaining a healthy anagen phase. Nutrients such as biotin, vitamins A, C, D, and E, iron, and zinc support cell proliferation and hair growth. A deficiency in these nutrients can lead to weakened hair and a shorter anagen phase.

- **Scalp Health:** A healthy scalp environment promotes robust hair growth. Conditions such as dandruff, seborrheic dermatitis, and fungal infections can disrupt the anagen phase by causing inflammation and damage to the hair follicles.
- **Medical Conditions:** Certain medical conditions, such as hypothyroidism, can affect the anagen phase by altering hormonal levels and metabolism. Treating underlying health issues is essential for restoring normal hair growth.

2. Catagen Phase (Transition Phase)

The catagen phase is a short transitional period where hair growth stops, and the follicle prepares to enter the resting phase. Factors influencing this phase include:

- **Hormonal Changes:** Hormonal fluctuations can impact the timing and duration of the catagen phase. For example, abrupt hormonal shifts during pregnancy or menopause can trigger premature catagen, leading to increased hair shedding.
- **Stress:** Acute stress can induce a premature catagen phase, causing a significant number of hairs to stop growing and enter the resting phase simultaneously. This condition, known as telogen effluvium, results in noticeable hair shedding.
- **Medical Treatments:** Certain medications and treatments, such as chemotherapy, can induce a rapid transition from anagen to catagen, leading to widespread hair loss. This effect is usually temporary, and hair growth resumes once the treatment is completed.

3. Telogen Phase (Resting Phase)

The telogen phase is the resting period where hair remains dormant before shedding. Factors affecting this phase include:

- **Nutritional Deficiencies:** Lack of essential nutrients can prolong the telogen phase, delaying the return to the anagen phase. Ensuring a balanced diet rich in vitamins and minerals supports timely hair renewal.
- **Chronic Stress:** Prolonged stress can extend the telogen phase, resulting in increased hair shedding and reduced hair density. Managing stress through relaxation techniques, exercise, and adequate sleep can help mitigate this effect.
- **Aging:** As people age, the duration of the telogen phase tends to increase, while the anagen phase shortens. This change leads to thinner hair and slower growth over time. Adopting healthy lifestyle practices can help mitigate age-related changes.
- **Seasonal Changes:** Research suggests that seasonal variations can influence the telogen phase. For instance, some individuals may experience increased hair shedding in the late summer and early fall due to changes in daylight and temperature.

4. Exogen Phase (Shedding Phase)

The exogen phase involves the shedding of old hair and the emergence of new hair. Factors influencing this phase include:

- **Scalp Health:** Conditions such as scalp psoriasis or eczema can disrupt the exogen phase, causing irregular shedding patterns. Maintaining a healthy scalp through proper hygiene and treatment of skin conditions supports normal hair shedding.
- **Hair Care Practices:** Harsh hair care practices, such as excessive brushing, tight hairstyles, and the use of chemical treatments, can accelerate hair shedding during the exogen phase. Gentle handling and the use of mild, natural hair care products can reduce mechanical stress on the hair.
- **Hormonal Imbalances:** Hormonal imbalances, particularly involving thyroid hormones and sex hormones, can affect the exogen phase. Addressing underlying hormonal issues through medical intervention can help regulate hair shedding.

Factors Affecting Hair Growth

Internal and external factors

Hair growth is influenced by a myriad of internal and external factors. Understanding these factors is crucial for developing an effective hair care routine and addressing issues related to hair health. Here, we explore the internal and external factors that play significant roles in hair growth.

Internal Factors

1. Genetics

- **Hereditary Influence:** Genetics is one of the primary determinants of hair growth patterns, hair density, and hair color. Hereditary conditions such as androgenetic alopecia (pattern baldness) can significantly influence hair growth, leading to thinning hair and baldness in both men and women.
- **Growth Cycle Duration:** Genetic factors determine the length of the anagen (growth) phase of the hair cycle, which in turn affects how long hair can grow. Individuals with longer anagen phases can grow their hair longer than those with shorter phases.

2. Hormonal Balance

- **Androgens:** Androgens, particularly dihydrotestosterone (DHT), play a crucial role in hair growth. High levels of DHT can shrink hair follicles and shorten the hair growth cycle, leading to thinning hair and hair loss, especially in individuals genetically predisposed to androgenetic alopecia.
- **Thyroid Hormones:** Thyroid hormones regulate metabolism and influence hair growth. Both hyperthyroidism (overactive thyroid) and hypothyroidism (underactive thyroid) can cause hair thinning and hair loss.
- **Sex Hormones:** Hormonal changes due to pregnancy, menopause, or hormonal imbalances can affect hair growth. For example, many women experience increased hair growth during pregnancy due to elevated estrogen levels, followed by postpartum hair shedding as hormone levels normalize.

3. Nutrition

- **Vitamins and Minerals:** Adequate intake of essential vitamins and minerals is vital for healthy hair growth. Nutrients such as biotin, vitamin D, vitamin E, iron, and zinc support hair follicle function and hair shaft production. Deficiencies in these nutrients can lead to weakened hair and increased hair shedding.
- **Proteins:** Hair is primarily composed of keratin, a protein. Adequate protein intake is essential for the production and maintenance of strong, healthy hair. A diet lacking in protein can result in brittle hair and slowed hair growth.

4. Overall Health

- **Chronic Illnesses:** Certain chronic illnesses, such as diabetes, lupus, and autoimmune diseases, can affect hair growth by disrupting the body's normal physiological processes.
- **Medications:** Some medications, including those for cancer treatment (chemotherapy), blood pressure, and depression, can have side effects that include hair loss. Understanding these side effects can help in managing hair health while on medication.

External Factors

1. Environmental Exposure

- **UV Radiation:** Prolonged exposure to ultraviolet (UV) radiation from the sun can damage the hair shaft and weaken the hair, making it more prone to breakage and split ends. Wearing hats or using hair products with UV protection can help mitigate this damage.
- **Pollution:** Air pollution can deposit harmful particles on the scalp and hair, leading to oxidative stress and inflammation. These conditions can weaken hair follicles and contribute to hair loss. Regular cleansing and protective measures can reduce the impact of pollution on hair.

2. Hair Care Practices

- **Chemical Treatments:** Frequent use of chemical treatments such as coloring, perming, and relaxing can damage the hair shaft and weaken the hair. These treatments can strip the hair of its natural oils, leading to dryness and brittleness.
- **Heat Styling:** Excessive use of heat styling tools like blow dryers, curling irons, and straighteners can cause heat damage to the hair shaft. This damage leads to moisture loss, split ends, and breakage. Using heat protectant products and limiting heat styling can help protect hair.
- **Tight Hairstyles:** Wearing tight hairstyles, such as ponytails, braids, and buns, can put excessive tension on the hair follicles, leading to a condition called traction alopecia. This condition can cause hair to break and fall out. Alternating hairstyles and avoiding tight styles can prevent this type of hair loss.

3. Scalp Health

- **Hygiene:** Proper scalp hygiene is essential for healthy hair growth. Regular washing removes excess oil, dead skin cells, and product buildup that can clog hair follicles and inhibit growth. Using gentle, natural shampoos can help maintain a clean and healthy scalp.
- **Scalp Conditions:** Conditions such as dandruff, psoriasis, and seborrheic dermatitis can affect hair growth by causing inflammation and irritation of the scalp. Treating these conditions with appropriate medicated shampoos and topical treatments is crucial for maintaining a healthy scalp environment.

4. Stress and Lifestyle

- **Stress:** Chronic stress can lead to hair loss conditions such as telogen effluvium, where a large number of hair follicles enter the telogen (resting) phase prematurely, resulting in noticeable hair shedding. Managing stress through relaxation techniques, exercise, and adequate sleep is vital for healthy hair growth.
- **Sleep:** Adequate sleep is essential for overall health and well-being, including hair health. Poor sleep can disrupt the body's natural growth and repair processes, including hair growth. Ensuring sufficient rest supports optimal hair health.

Impact of lifestyle and environment

Hair growth is not only a reflection of genetic predisposition and internal health but also significantly influenced by lifestyle choices and environmental factors. Understanding the impact of these elements can help in crafting a holistic approach to hair care that promotes optimal growth and health. Here, we explore how various lifestyle habits and environmental conditions affect hair growth and overall hair health.

Lifestyle Factors

1. Nutrition and Diet

- **Balanced Diet:** A diet rich in essential nutrients supports the health of hair follicles and the hair growth cycle. Vitamins, minerals, and proteins are crucial for the formation and maintenance of healthy hair. Consuming a variety of fruits, vegetables, lean proteins, and whole grains ensures that your body gets the nutrients it needs for robust hair growth.
- **Specific Nutrients:** Certain nutrients are particularly important for hair health:
  - **Biotin (Vitamin B7):** Promotes hair strength and growth by aiding in the production of keratin.
  - **Vitamin D:** Essential for hair follicle cycling and preventing hair loss.
  - **Iron:** Prevents hair loss by supporting the production of hemoglobin, which carries oxygen to the hair follicles.
  - **Zinc:** Vital for hair tissue growth and repair.
  - **Omega-3 Fatty Acids:** Promote scalp health and hair hydration.

2. Hydration

- **Water Intake:** Adequate hydration is essential for overall health, including hair health. Drinking sufficient water ensures that hair follicles remain hydrated, which is crucial for hair growth and strength. Dehydration can lead to dry, brittle hair that is prone to breakage.

3. Physical Activity

- **Exercise:** Regular physical activity promotes overall health and well-being, which indirectly benefits hair growth. Exercise improves blood circulation, ensuring that hair follicles receive an adequate supply of oxygen and nutrients. It also helps reduce stress levels, which can have a positive impact on hair growth.

4. Stress Management

- **Chronic Stress:** Persistent stress can disrupt the hair growth cycle, leading to conditions such as telogen effluvium, where a large number of hair follicles enter the resting phase prematurely, resulting in increased hair shedding. Stress management techniques such as yoga, meditation, deep breathing exercises, and adequate sleep can help mitigate the negative effects of stress on hair health.
- **Sleep Quality:** Quality sleep is crucial for the body's repair and regeneration processes, including hair growth. Poor sleep can disrupt hormonal balance and impair the body's ability to repair hair follicles, leading to weakened hair and increased shedding.

5. Hair Care Practices

- **Gentle Handling:** Treating hair gently during washing, drying, and styling can prevent damage. Using wide-toothed combs, avoiding excessive brushing, and limiting the use of heat styling tools help maintain hair integrity.
- **Product Choices:** Choosing natural, sulfate-free shampoos and conditioners can reduce exposure to harsh chemicals that strip the hair of natural oils. Products containing nourishing ingredients like aloe vera, coconut oil, and castor oil support hair health.

Environmental Factors

1. Sun Exposure

- **UV Radiation:** Prolonged exposure to ultraviolet (UV) radiation from the sun can damage the hair cuticle and weaken the hair shaft, leading to dryness, brittleness, and increased risk of split ends. Wearing hats or using hair products with UV protection can help shield hair from sun damage.

2. Pollution

- **Air Pollution:** Pollutants such as dust, smoke, and industrial emissions can settle on the scalp and hair, causing oxidative stress and inflammation. These factors can weaken hair follicles and impair hair growth. Regular cleansing with mild shampoos can help remove pollutants and protect hair health.

3. Climate and Weather

- **Humidity:** High humidity levels can cause hair to absorb moisture from the air, leading to frizz and breakage. Using anti-frizz products and protective hairstyles can help manage humidity-related issues.
- **Dry Air:** In contrast, dry air, especially during winter, can strip hair of its natural moisture, leading to dryness and brittleness. Using humidifiers indoors and moisturizing hair care products can help maintain hydration.

4. Water Quality

- **Hard Water:** Water with high mineral content (hard water) can leave residues on the hair and scalp, making hair feel dry and look dull. Using a clarifying shampoo or installing a water softener can help mitigate the effects of hard water on hair.

5. Chemicals and Toxins

- **Chemical Exposure:** Frequent exposure to chlorine (in swimming pools) and other chemicals can damage the hair cuticle, leading to dryness and breakage. Rinsing hair after swimming and using protective hair products can help minimize chemical damage.

Conclusion

Lifestyle choices and environmental conditions play significant roles in determining the health and growth of hair. By adopting a balanced diet, staying hydrated, managing stress, engaging in regular physical activity, and practicing gentle hair care, you can support optimal hair growth. Additionally, protecting your hair from environmental damage through proper hygiene, protective styling, and the use of suitable hair care products will help maintain healthy, resilient hair. Understanding these factors empowers you to take a proactive approach to hair care, ensuring that your hair remains strong, vibrant, and beautiful.

Common Hair Problems

Hair Loss

Types of hair loss

Hair loss is a common concern affecting millions of people worldwide. It can be caused by a variety of factors, including genetics, hormonal changes, medical conditions, and lifestyle choices. Understanding the different types of hair loss is essential for identifying the underlying causes and seeking appropriate treatments. Here, we explore the most common types of hair loss.

1. Androgenetic Alopecia (Pattern Baldness)

- **Overview:** Androgenetic alopecia, commonly known as pattern baldness, is the most prevalent type of hair loss. It affects both men and women and is primarily driven by genetic and hormonal factors.
- **Male Pattern Baldness:** In men, androgenetic alopecia typically presents as a receding hairline and thinning at the crown. Over time, these areas may merge, leading to complete baldness on the top of the head while the sides and back remain unaffected.
- **Female Pattern Baldness:** Women with androgenetic alopecia usually experience diffuse thinning across the crown with the frontal hairline remaining intact. Complete baldness is rare in women.
- **Causes:** Androgenetic alopecia is caused by a combination of genetic predisposition and the influence of androgens (male hormones), particularly dihydrotestosterone (DHT). DHT binds to hair follicles, causing them to shrink and produce thinner, shorter hairs.

2. Telogen Effluvium

- **Overview:** Telogen effluvium is a temporary form of hair loss characterized by widespread thinning or shedding of hair. It occurs when a significant number of hair follicles enter the telogen (resting) phase prematurely.
- **Causes:** Common triggers include physical or emotional stress, surgery, severe illness, drastic weight loss, or hormonal changes such as those experienced postpartum. Nutritional deficiencies and certain medications can also induce telogen effluvium.
- **Symptoms:** The primary symptom is diffuse thinning of hair across the scalp, often noticeable when washing or brushing the hair. Unlike androgenetic alopecia, telogen effluvium does not usually cause complete baldness.

3. Alopecia Areata

- **Overview:** Alopecia areata is an autoimmune condition that causes patchy hair loss. The body's immune system mistakenly attacks hair follicles, resulting in hair falling out in small, round patches.
- **Types:** Alopecia areata can progress to alopecia totalis (complete loss of scalp hair) or alopecia universalis (complete loss of all body hair), though these cases are rare.
- **Causes:** The exact cause of alopecia areata is unknown, but it is believed to involve a combination of genetic predisposition and environmental triggers. Stress and viral infections are potential triggers.
- **Symptoms:** The hallmark of alopecia areata is the sudden appearance of round, smooth patches of hair loss. In some cases, nail changes such as pitting or ridging may also occur.

4. Traction Alopecia

- **Overview:** Traction alopecia is caused by prolonged tension on the hair, usually from tight hairstyles. It is common in individuals who frequently wear braids, ponytails, buns, or extensions.
- **Causes:** The constant pulling force on the hair follicles leads to inflammation and damage, which can eventually result in permanent hair loss if not addressed.
- **Symptoms:** Early signs include redness, bumps, and folliculitis (inflammation of hair follicles) along the hairline or areas under tension. Over time, hair in these areas thins and may stop growing entirely.

5. Anagen Effluvium

- **Overview:** Anagen effluvium is rapid hair loss resulting from an interruption in the anagen (growth) phase of the hair cycle. It is most commonly associated with chemotherapy and radiation treatments for cancer.
- **Causes:** The treatment targets rapidly dividing cells, including those in the hair follicles, leading to sudden hair loss.
- **Symptoms:** Hair loss begins within days to weeks of starting treatment and can affect hair on the scalp, as well as body hair, eyebrows, and eyelashes.

6. Cicatricial (Scarring) Alopecia

- **Overview:** Cicatricial alopecia, also known as scarring alopecia, is a group of rare disorders that destroy hair follicles and replace them with scar tissue, leading to permanent hair loss.
- **Types:** This condition can be primary (where the hair follicle is the target of the disease) or secondary (where the follicle is destroyed by an external factor such as infection or injury).
- **Causes:** Causes vary and may include autoimmune diseases, infections, inflammatory conditions, and traumatic injuries. Examples include lichen planopilaris and frontal fibrosing alopecia.
- **Symptoms:** Symptoms include redness, swelling, pain, and hair loss in the affected area. Over time, the scalp may appear smooth and shiny where hair follicles have been destroyed.

7. Diffuse Alopecia

- **Overview:** Diffuse alopecia refers to a general thinning of hair across the entire scalp, without distinct patches or bald spots. It can be a symptom of underlying conditions or the result of environmental factors.
- **Causes:** Potential causes include nutritional deficiencies, hormonal imbalances, chronic illness, and exposure to toxins. Certain medications and treatments can also cause diffuse hair loss.
- **Symptoms:** Hair appears uniformly thin across the scalp, and there may be increased shedding when washing or brushing hair.

Understanding the various types of hair loss is essential for identifying the underlying causes and seeking appropriate treatment. Each type of hair loss has distinct characteristics and requires different approaches for management and recovery. By recognizing the symptoms and factors contributing to hair loss, individuals can take proactive steps to address their hair health concerns and seek professional guidance when necessary.

Causes and prevention

Hair loss can be distressing, but understanding its causes and prevention strategies can help manage and mitigate the issue. Various factors contribute to hair loss, including genetics, hormonal changes, medical conditions, and lifestyle choices. Here, we explore the common causes of hair loss and provide actionable prevention tips.

1. Androgenetic Alopecia (Pattern Baldness)

Causes:

- **Genetic Predisposition:** Androgenetic alopecia is primarily hereditary. If you have a family history of pattern baldness, you are more likely to experience it.
- **Hormonal Changes:** The presence of androgens, particularly dihydrotestosterone (DHT), plays a significant role. DHT binds to hair follicles, causing them to shrink and produce thinner, shorter hairs.

Prevention:

- **Minoxidil:** Over-the-counter topical treatments like minoxidil can slow hair loss and stimulate hair growth.
- **Finasteride:** Prescription medications such as finasteride can reduce DHT levels and prevent further hair loss.
- **Healthy Lifestyle:** Maintaining a balanced diet, regular exercise, and stress management can support overall hair health and potentially slow the progression of androgenetic alopecia.

2. Telogen Effluvium

Causes:

- **Physical or Emotional Stress:** Events such as surgery, severe illness, or significant life changes can trigger telogen effluvium.
- **Nutritional Deficiencies:** Lack of essential nutrients like iron, zinc, and vitamins can lead to hair shedding.
- **Hormonal Changes:** Postpartum women often experience telogen effluvium due to hormonal fluctuations after childbirth.

Prevention:

- **Balanced Diet:** Ensure adequate intake of vitamins and minerals to support hair health. Foods rich in iron, zinc, biotin, and vitamins A, C, D, and E are beneficial.
- **Stress Management:** Techniques such as meditation, yoga, and regular physical activity can help manage stress levels and reduce the risk of telogen effluvium.
- **Medical Advice:** Consult a healthcare provider for appropriate treatment if hormonal imbalances or medical conditions are the cause.

3. Alopecia Areata

Causes:

- **Autoimmune Disorder:** Alopecia areata occurs when the immune system mistakenly attacks hair follicles, leading to hair loss.
- **Genetic and Environmental Factors:** A combination of genetic predisposition and environmental triggers such as viral infections may contribute.

Prevention:

- **Corticosteroids:** Topical or injectable corticosteroids can reduce inflammation and promote hair regrowth.
- **Immunotherapy:** Treatments that modulate the immune response can help manage alopecia areata.
- **Supportive Care:** Maintaining a healthy lifestyle and managing stress can support overall immune health and potentially reduce flare-ups.

4. Traction Alopecia

Causes:

- **Tight Hairstyles:** Frequent use of tight hairstyles like braids, ponytails, and buns can cause traction alopecia.
- **Hair Extensions:** Continuous use of hair extensions that pull on the hair can lead to follicle damage and hair loss.

Prevention:

- **Loose Hairstyles:** Opt for looser hairstyles that do not put excessive tension on the hair and scalp.
- **Avoid Frequent Styling:** Give your hair breaks from tight styles and extensions to allow follicles to recover.
- **Protective Styles:** Use protective hairstyles that minimize stress on the hair, such as loose braids or twists.

5. Anagen Effluvium

Causes:

- **Chemotherapy and Radiation:** Treatments for cancer that target rapidly dividing cells, including hair follicle cells, cause anagen effluvium.
- **Toxic Exposure:** Exposure to certain toxins and chemicals can disrupt the anagen phase, leading to hair loss.

Prevention:

- **Scalp Cooling:** During chemotherapy, scalp cooling caps can help reduce hair loss by constricting blood vessels and minimizing the amount of chemotherapy reaching hair follicles.
- **Gentle Hair Care:** Use mild shampoos and avoid harsh treatments to reduce additional stress on hair.
- **Nutritional Support:** Ensure adequate nutrition to support overall health during cancer treatment.

6. Cicatricial (Scarring) Alopecia

Causes:

- **Autoimmune Diseases:** Conditions like lupus and lichen planopilaris can lead to scarring alopecia.
- **Infections and Inflammatory Conditions:** Severe infections and inflammatory scalp conditions can destroy hair follicles and replace them with scar tissue.

Prevention:

- **Early Diagnosis and Treatment:** Prompt treatment of underlying conditions with anti-inflammatory and antimicrobial medications can prevent progression.
- **Gentle Hair Care:** Avoid aggressive hair treatments that can exacerbate inflammation and damage.
- **Regular Monitoring:** Regular check-ups with a dermatologist can help manage the condition and prevent further scarring.

7. Diffuse Alopecia

Causes:

- **Nutritional Deficiencies:** Lack of essential nutrients can cause diffuse hair thinning.
- **Hormonal Imbalances:** Conditions like hypothyroidism and polycystic ovary syndrome (PCOS) can lead to diffuse alopecia.
- **Chronic Illnesses:** Long-term illnesses can affect overall hair health and growth.

Prevention:

- **Nutrient-Rich Diet:** Consuming a balanced diet with sufficient vitamins and minerals supports hair health.
- **Medical Management:** Addressing underlying hormonal imbalances or chronic illnesses with appropriate medical treatment is crucial.
- **Healthy Lifestyle:** Regular exercise, adequate sleep, and stress management contribute to overall health and support hair growth.

Conclusion

Hair loss can stem from various causes, each requiring specific prevention and treatment strategies. Understanding the underlying factors contributing to hair loss is essential for developing an effective approach to manage and mitigate its effects. By adopting a healthy lifestyle, seeking appropriate medical advice, and practicing gentle hair care, you can support your hair's health and potentially prevent further hair loss.

Thinning Hair

Reasons behind thinning hair

Thinning hair is a widespread concern that can affect individuals of all ages and genders. It occurs when the density of hair decreases, leading to a less voluminous appearance. Understanding the reasons behind thinning hair is crucial for developing effective strategies to address this issue. Here, we explore the primary factors that contribute to hair thinning.

1. Genetic Factors

- **Androgenetic Alopecia:** The most common cause of thinning hair is androgenetic alopecia, also known as male or female pattern baldness. This hereditary condition is influenced by genetic predisposition and hormonal factors. In men, it typically presents as a receding hairline and thinning at the crown, while in women, it manifests as diffuse thinning across the scalp.
- **Family History:** If you have a family history of thinning hair or pattern baldness, you are more likely to experience similar hair loss patterns.

2. Hormonal Changes

- **Menopause:** Women often experience thinning hair during menopause due to a decline in estrogen levels. Estrogen helps to keep hair in the anagen (growth) phase for longer periods, so reduced levels can lead to shorter growth cycles and increased hair shedding.
- **Pregnancy and Postpartum:** Hormonal fluctuations during pregnancy can lead to thicker hair, but many women experience significant shedding (telogen effluvium) postpartum as hormone levels normalize.
- **Thyroid Imbalance:** Both hyperthyroidism (overactive thyroid) and hypothyroidism (underactive thyroid) can cause hair thinning. Thyroid hormones play a vital role in regulating the hair growth cycle.

3. Nutritional Deficiencies

- **Iron Deficiency:** Iron is essential for producing hemoglobin, which carries oxygen to the hair follicles. A lack of iron can lead to anemia and subsequent hair thinning.
- **Vitamin Deficiencies:** Deficiencies in vitamins such as biotin (B7), vitamin D, vitamin E, and vitamin A can impair hair growth and contribute to thinning. These vitamins are crucial for maintaining healthy hair follicles and promoting growth.
- **Protein Deficiency:** Hair is primarily composed of keratin, a protein. Inadequate protein intake can result in weakened hair shafts and increased hair loss.

4. Stress

- **Physical and Emotional Stress:** Significant physical or emotional stress can trigger telogen effluvium, a condition where a large number of hair follicles enter the telogen (resting) phase prematurely. This leads to noticeable hair shedding and thinning.
- **Chronic Stress:** Prolonged stress can disrupt the hair growth cycle, leading to persistent thinning. Stress management techniques such as meditation, exercise, and adequate sleep can help mitigate this effect.

5. Medical Conditions

- **Autoimmune Diseases:** Conditions such as alopecia areata, lupus, and lichen planopilaris can cause thinning hair. In these conditions, the immune system mistakenly attacks hair follicles, leading to hair loss.
- **Scalp Infections:** Fungal infections like ringworm can cause localized hair thinning and patchy hair loss. Treating the underlying infection is essential for restoring hair growth.

6. Medications and Treatments

- **Chemotherapy:** Chemotherapy drugs target rapidly dividing cells, including those in hair follicles. This can lead to sudden and significant hair thinning or loss.
- **Medications:** Certain medications, including those for blood pressure, depression, and heart conditions, can have side effects that include hair thinning. If you suspect your medication is affecting your hair, consult your doctor for possible alternatives.

7. Environmental Factors

- **Pollution:** Environmental pollutants can damage the scalp and hair, leading to weakened hair follicles and thinning. Regular cleansing and using protective hair products can help mitigate this damage.
- **UV Radiation:** Prolonged exposure to ultraviolet (UV) radiation from the sun can weaken hair and cause thinning. Wearing hats or using hair products with UV protection can help shield your hair from sun damage.

8. Hair Care Practices

- **Chemical Treatments:** Frequent use of chemical treatments such as coloring, perming, and relaxing can damage the hair shaft and follicles, leading to thinning hair.
- **Heat Styling:** Excessive use of heat styling tools like blow dryers, curling irons, and straighteners can cause heat damage to the hair, resulting in dryness and breakage.
- **Tight Hairstyles:** Wearing tight hairstyles such as ponytails, braids, and buns can cause traction alopecia, a condition where constant pulling leads to hair thinning and loss.

9. Aging

- **Natural Aging Process:** As we age, hair naturally becomes thinner due to a decrease in the number of active hair follicles. The growth rate of hair also slows down, and the hair shaft itself may become finer.
- **Hormonal Changes:** Age-related hormonal changes can contribute to thinning hair. For example, decreased levels of estrogen and progesterone in women during menopause can lead to thinner hair.

Treatment options

Thinning hair can be a source of distress, but there are numerous treatment options available that can help address the issue. The choice of treatment depends on the underlying cause of hair thinning. Here, we explore various treatment options, ranging from lifestyle changes and natural remedies to medical treatments and advanced hair restoration techniques.

1. Lifestyle Changes

Diet and Nutrition:

- **Balanced Diet:** Ensure a diet rich in essential nutrients such as vitamins (A, C, D, E, and B-complex), minerals (iron, zinc), and proteins to support hair health.
- **Hydration:** Drink plenty of water to keep hair hydrated and maintain overall health.

- **Supplements:** Consider supplements if dietary intake is insufficient, especially biotin, iron, vitamin D, and omega-3 fatty acids. Consult with a healthcare provider before starting any new supplements.

Stress Management:

- **Relaxation Techniques:** Practices such as yoga, meditation, and deep breathing exercises can help manage stress levels, which in turn can reduce hair thinning.
- **Exercise:** Regular physical activity improves overall health and reduces stress, promoting a healthy hair growth cycle.

Sleep Hygiene:

- **Adequate Sleep:** Ensure you get 7-8 hours of quality sleep per night to support the body's repair and regeneration processes, including hair growth.

2. Hair Care Practices

Gentle Handling:

- **Avoid Over-Styling:** Minimize the use of heat styling tools and chemical treatments that can damage hair.
- **Protective Hairstyles:** Opt for loose hairstyles that do not put excessive tension on the hair and scalp.

Appropriate Hair Products:

- **Sulfate-Free Shampoos:** Use gentle, sulfate-free shampoos that do not strip hair of its natural oils.
- **Conditioners and Masks:** Regularly use conditioners and deep-conditioning masks to keep hair moisturized and nourished.
- **Scalp Treatments:** Use products specifically designed to improve scalp health, such as those containing tea tree oil, salicylic acid, or ketoconazole.

3. Topical Treatments

Minoxidil:

- **Overview:** Minoxidil is an over-the-counter topical treatment approved by the FDA for treating hair thinning and loss.
- **Usage:** Apply minoxidil solution or foam to the scalp twice daily to stimulate hair growth and slow down hair loss.
- **Effectiveness:** Results may take several months to become noticeable, and continuous use is necessary to maintain benefits.

Natural Oils:

- **Castor Oil:** Known for its ability to promote hair growth, castor oil can be massaged into the scalp to improve circulation and nourish hair follicles.

- **Essential Oils:** Oils like rosemary, peppermint, and lavender have shown potential in promoting hair growth. They can be mixed with carrier oils and applied to the scalp.

4. Oral Medications

Finasteride:

- **Overview:** Finasteride is a prescription medication that inhibits the conversion of testosterone to dihydrotestosterone (DHT), a hormone linked to hair thinning and loss.
- **Usage:** Taken orally, finasteride is primarily used for male pattern baldness.
- **Effectiveness:** Regular use can reduce hair loss and promote regrowth, but it may take several months to see results. It is not recommended for use by women, especially during pregnancy.

Spironolactone:

- **Overview:** Spironolactone is an anti-androgen medication that can be used to treat hair thinning in women with hormonal imbalances.
- **Usage:** Taken orally, it helps reduce androgen levels, which can contribute to hair thinning.
- **Effectiveness:** It can be effective in treating female pattern hair loss, particularly in those with conditions like polycystic ovary syndrome (PCOS).

5. Medical Treatments

Platelet-Rich Plasma (PRP) Therapy:

- **Overview:** PRP therapy involves drawing a patient's blood, processing it to concentrate the platelets, and then injecting it into the scalp.
- **Mechanism:** Platelets contain growth factors that can stimulate hair follicle activity and promote new hair growth.
- **Effectiveness:** PRP therapy has shown promise in treating hair thinning, but results can vary. Multiple sessions are usually required.

Low-Level Laser Therapy (LLLT):

- **Overview:** LLLT uses red light or near-infrared light to stimulate hair follicles and promote hair growth.
- **Mechanism:** The light therapy increases blood flow to the scalp and energizes hair follicles.
- **Effectiveness:** LLLT can be effective for some individuals, especially when used in conjunction with other treatments like minoxidil or finasteride.

6. Advanced Hair Restoration Techniques

Hair Transplant Surgery:

- **Overview:** Hair transplant surgery involves moving hair follicles from one part of the scalp (donor site) to the thinning or balding areas (recipient site).
- **Techniques:** Common techniques include Follicular Unit Transplantation (FUT) and Follicular Unit Extraction (FUE).
- **Effectiveness:** Hair transplant surgery can provide permanent and natural-looking results, but it is a more invasive and expensive option.

Scalp Micropigmentation (SMP):

- **Overview:** SMP is a non-surgical procedure that uses tiny pigment deposits to create the appearance of fuller hair or a closely-shaved scalp.
- **Mechanism:** The procedure mimics the look of hair follicles, providing the illusion of density.
- **Effectiveness:** SMP can be a good option for those who prefer a low-maintenance solution and do not want surgery.

Thinning hair can be addressed through a variety of treatment options, from lifestyle changes and natural remedies to medical treatments and advanced hair restoration techniques. The choice of treatment depends on the underlying cause of hair thinning and individual preferences. Consulting with a healthcare provider or a dermatologist can help determine the most appropriate treatment plan for your specific needs. By taking a comprehensive approach to hair care, you can improve hair density, strength, and overall health.

Damaged Hair

Causes of hair damage

Hair damage is a prevalent issue that can affect individuals of all ages. Damaged hair is characterized by a rough texture, dryness, split ends, and breakage. Understanding the causes of hair damage is essential for developing effective prevention and treatment strategies. Here, we explore the primary factors that contribute to hair damage.

1. Chemical Treatments

Hair Coloring:

- **Bleaching:** Bleaching hair to achieve lighter colors involves the use of strong chemicals that strip the hair of its natural pigment. This process breaks down the hair's structure, leading to dryness, brittleness, and increased susceptibility to damage.

- **Dyeing:** Regular use of hair dyes, especially permanent dyes, can weaken the hair shaft and cause damage over time. The chemicals in dyes penetrate the hair cuticle, altering its structure and leading to potential damage.

Perming and Relaxing:

- **Perming:** Perming involves using chemicals to break and reform the bonds in hair, creating curls or waves. This process can weaken the hair's structure, making it prone to breakage and split ends.
- **Relaxing:** Relaxers use strong chemicals to straighten curly or wavy hair by breaking down the hair's natural structure. Frequent use of relaxers can lead to severe damage, including hair thinning and breakage.

2. Heat Styling

Blow Drying:

- **High Heat:** Regular use of blow dryers at high temperatures can strip hair of its natural moisture, leading to dryness and brittleness. The intense heat can weaken the hair shaft, causing breakage.

Flat Irons and Curling Irons:

- **Direct Heat:** Flat irons and curling irons apply direct heat to the hair, which can damage the cuticle and lead to split ends and breakage. Frequent use without proper heat protection can exacerbate damage.

3. Mechanical Damage

Brushing and Combing:

- **Excessive Brushing:** Over-brushing or using brushes with harsh bristles can cause physical damage to the hair shaft, leading to split ends and breakage.
- **Wet Hair:** Brushing or combing hair when it is wet and more elastic can cause stretching and breakage. It is recommended to use a wide-toothed comb and be gentle with wet hair.

Tight Hairstyles:

- **Ponytails and Buns:** Wearing tight ponytails, buns, or braids can put excessive tension on the hair, leading to breakage and traction alopecia (hair loss due to pulling).
- **Hair Accessories:** Using hair ties, clips, and pins that are too tight or have rough edges can cause mechanical damage to the hair shaft.

4. Environmental Factors

Sun Exposure:

- **UV Radiation:** Prolonged exposure to ultraviolet (UV) radiation from the sun can weaken the hair cuticle and cause color fading, dryness, and brittleness. UV rays can break down the protein structure of hair, making it more susceptible to damage.

Pollution:

- **Air Pollutants:** Environmental pollutants such as dust, smoke, and chemicals can settle on the hair and scalp, leading to oxidative stress and damage. These pollutants can weaken the hair shaft and make it more prone to breakage.

Chlorine and Saltwater:

- **Swimming:** Chlorine in swimming pools and saltwater from the ocean can strip hair of its natural oils, leading to dryness and brittleness. Both chlorine and salt can cause the hair cuticle to lift, increasing the risk of damage.

5. Lack of Proper Hair Care

Infrequent Trimming:

- **Split Ends:** Not trimming hair regularly can lead to the development of split ends, which can travel up the hair shaft and cause further breakage. Regular trims help maintain healthy hair and prevent damage from spreading.

Improper Washing:

- **Harsh Shampoos:** Using shampoos with sulfates and other harsh chemicals can strip the hair of its natural oils, leading to dryness and damage. It is essential to use gentle, sulfate-free shampoos to maintain hair health.
- **Over-Washing:** Washing hair too frequently can remove natural oils, leading to dryness and increased susceptibility to damage. It is recommended to wash hair according to its specific needs and type.

6. Nutritional Deficiencies

Inadequate Nutrition:

- **Essential Nutrients:** A lack of essential nutrients, such as vitamins (A, C, D, E, and B-complex), minerals (iron, zinc), and proteins, can weaken the hair and make it more prone to damage. A balanced diet is crucial for maintaining strong, healthy hair.

7. Medical Conditions

Hormonal Imbalances:

- **Thyroid Disorders:** Conditions such as hypothyroidism and hyperthyroidism can affect the health of hair, making it dry, brittle, and more prone to breakage.
- **PCOS:** Polycystic ovary syndrome (PCOS) and other hormonal imbalances can lead to changes in hair texture and health, resulting in damage and thinning.

Repair and prevention strategies

Addressing hair damage requires a combination of effective repair and prevention strategies. By understanding the underlying causes of hair damage and implementing targeted solutions, you can restore hair health and prevent further damage. Here, we explore various strategies to repair damaged hair and prevent future damage.

1. Repair Strategies

Deep Conditioning Treatments:

- **Hair Masks:** Use deep conditioning hair masks at least once a week to provide intense hydration and nourishment. Look for masks containing ingredients like shea butter, coconut oil, and keratin, which help repair and strengthen damaged hair.
- **Leave-In Conditioners:** Apply leave-in conditioners to provide ongoing moisture and protection throughout the day. These products help seal the cuticle and reduce frizz.

Protein Treatments:

- **Reconstructive Treatments:** Use protein-based treatments to rebuild and strengthen the hair shaft. These treatments can help repair the damage caused by chemical treatments and heat styling.
- **Hydrolyzed Proteins:** Look for products containing hydrolyzed proteins, which can penetrate the hair shaft and reinforce its structure.

Trim Regularly:

- **Split End Trimming:** Regular trims every 6-8 weeks help remove split ends and prevent them from traveling up the hair shaft, reducing breakage and maintaining healthy hair.

Scalp Care:

- **Scalp Massages:** Regular scalp massages with nourishing oils, such as castor oil or jojoba oil, can improve blood circulation, promote hair growth, and maintain scalp health.
- **Scalp Treatments:** Use treatments that address specific scalp issues, such as dandruff or dryness. Ingredients like tea tree oil, salicylic acid, and zinc pyrithione can help maintain a healthy scalp environment.

Heat Protection:

- **Heat Protectant Sprays:** Before using heat styling tools, apply a heat protectant spray to shield hair from high temperatures and prevent damage.
- **Lower Heat Settings:** Use the lowest effective heat setting on styling tools to minimize damage.

Natural Oils:

- **Coconut Oil:** Known for its penetrating properties, coconut oil can be used as a pre-shampoo treatment to reduce protein loss and strengthen hair.
- **Argan Oil:** Apply argan oil to the hair to add shine, reduce frizz, and protect against environmental damage.

2. Prevention Strategies

Gentle Hair Care Practices:

- **Avoid Over-Washing:** Washing hair too frequently can strip it of natural oils. Adjust your washing routine based on your hair type and condition.
- **Mild Shampoos:** Use sulfate-free shampoos and gentle cleansers to maintain the hair's natural moisture balance.
- **Condition Regularly:** Always use a conditioner after shampooing to restore moisture and protect the hair cuticle.

Protective Hairstyles:

- **Avoid Tight Styles:** Opt for loose hairstyles that do not put excessive tension on the hair and scalp. Tight ponytails, braids, and buns can cause mechanical damage and breakage.
- **Night Protection:** Use satin or silk pillowcases and hair wraps to reduce friction and prevent hair breakage while sleeping.

Limit Chemical Treatments:

- **Reduce Frequency:** Limit the use of chemical treatments like coloring, perming, and relaxing. When you do use these treatments, ensure they are spaced out to give your hair time to recover.
- **Professional Services:** Seek professional help for chemical treatments to ensure they are done correctly and with the least damage possible.

Heat Styling Precautions:

- **Air Drying:** Whenever possible, let your hair air dry instead of using a blow dryer. If you must use a blow dryer, choose a low heat setting and keep the dryer at a safe distance from your hair.
- **Heat Styling Alternatives:** Explore heat-free styling methods such as braiding, twisting, or using foam rollers to achieve your desired look without exposing your hair to high temperatures.

Environmental Protection:

- **UV Protection:** Use hair products with UV filters to protect your hair from sun damage. Wearing hats or scarves can also provide physical protection from the sun.
- **Chlorine and Saltwater:** Before swimming in a pool or the ocean, wet your hair and apply a leave-in conditioner or oil to create a protective barrier. After swimming, rinse your hair thoroughly to remove chlorine or salt.

Healthy Lifestyle Choices:

- **Balanced Diet:** Maintain a diet rich in vitamins, minerals, and proteins to support hair health from within. Foods like eggs, nuts, seeds, fish, and leafy greens are excellent for hair health.
- **Hydration:** Drink plenty of water to keep your hair hydrated and support overall health.
- **Regular Exercise:** Engage in regular physical activity to improve blood circulation, which benefits hair growth and health.

Avoid Over-Brushing:

- **Gentle Combing:** Use a wide-toothed comb to detangle wet hair gently. Avoid excessive brushing, which can cause mechanical damage and breakage.

Stress Management:

- **Relaxation Techniques:** Practice relaxation techniques such as yoga, meditation, and deep breathing exercises to manage stress levels, which can impact hair health.
- **Adequate Sleep:** Ensure you get 7-8 hours of quality sleep each night to support the body's repair and regeneration processes, including hair growth.

Natural Hair Care Basics

Benefits of Natural Hair Care

Advantages over synthetic products

Natural hair care is increasingly popular as people seek healthier, more sustainable ways to maintain and enhance their hair. Using natural ingredients and methods offers numerous benefits compared to synthetic products, which often contain harsh chemicals. Here, we explore the advantages of natural hair care and why it is a preferred choice for many.

1. Gentle on Hair and Scalp

Reduced Chemical Exposure:

- **No Harsh Chemicals:** Natural hair care products are free from harsh chemicals such as sulfates, parabens, and silicones, which can strip the hair of its natural oils and cause dryness and irritation.
- **Minimal Side Effects:** Natural ingredients are less likely to cause allergic reactions or scalp sensitivity compared to synthetic chemicals.

Moisturizing Properties:

- **Natural Oils:** Ingredients like coconut oil, argan oil, and shea butter provide deep hydration and nourishment, helping to maintain the hair's natural moisture balance.
- **Soothing Effect:** Natural products often contain soothing agents like aloe vera and chamomile, which can calm an irritated scalp and reduce inflammation.

2. Environmentally Friendly

Biodegradable Ingredients:

- **Eco-Friendly:** Natural hair care products typically use biodegradable ingredients that do not harm the environment when washed down the drain.
- **Sustainable Sourcing:** Many natural products are sourced sustainably, ensuring minimal impact on the environment and supporting ethical practices.

Reduced Pollution:

- **Less Packaging Waste:** Natural hair care brands often use eco-friendly packaging, such as recyclable or biodegradable materials, reducing environmental pollution.
- **Fewer Pollutants:** By avoiding synthetic chemicals, natural hair care reduces the release of pollutants into water systems and soil.

3. Supports Overall Hair Health

Nutrient-Rich Formulas:

- **Vitamins and Minerals:** Natural ingredients are rich in essential vitamins and minerals that support hair health, such as vitamin E, vitamin A, and biotin.
- **Proteins:** Many natural products contain proteins that strengthen the hair shaft and reduce breakage.

Scalp Health:

- **Balanced pH:** Natural products help maintain the scalp's natural pH balance, preventing issues like dandruff and dryness.
- **Antimicrobial Properties:** Ingredients like tea tree oil and peppermint oil have natural antimicrobial properties that can help combat scalp infections and promote a healthy scalp environment.

4. Long-Term Benefits

Strengthens Hair:

- **Less Breakage:** By avoiding harsh chemicals, natural hair care helps reduce hair breakage and split ends, leading to stronger, healthier hair over time.
- **Improves Elasticity:** Natural ingredients can improve hair elasticity, making it more resilient to styling and environmental stressors.

Enhances Shine:

- **Natural Luster:** Regular use of natural oils and conditioners can enhance the hair's natural shine and luster, giving it a healthy, vibrant appearance.

Promotes Hair Growth:

- **Stimulates Follicles:** Ingredients like castor oil, rosemary oil, and peppermint oil can stimulate hair follicles and promote hair growth.
- **Reduces Hair Loss:** Natural products can help reduce hair loss by strengthening the hair roots and minimizing damage from environmental factors.

5. Customizable and Versatile

DIY Options:

- **Homemade Recipes:** Natural hair care allows for creating customized hair treatments at home using readily available ingredients like honey, avocado, and yogurt.
- **Tailored Solutions:** DIY natural hair care recipes can be tailored to address specific hair concerns, such as dryness, frizz, or dandruff.

Multipurpose Uses:

- **Versatility:** Many natural ingredients can be used for multiple purposes, such as coconut oil for hair conditioning, skin moisturizing, and even cooking.
- **Cost-Effective:** Natural hair care can be more cost-effective in the long run, as many ingredients are affordable and have multiple uses.

6. Ethical and Cruelty-Free

Animal Welfare:

- **Cruelty-Free:** Many natural hair care brands prioritize cruelty-free practices, ensuring that their products are not tested on animals.
- **Vegan Options:** Natural hair care often includes vegan-friendly products, catering to consumers who prefer plant-based options.

Ethical Production:

- **Fair Trade:** Natural hair care brands often support fair trade practices, ensuring that the ingredients are sourced ethically and that workers are paid fairly.
- **Community Support:** Purchasing natural hair care products can support local communities and small businesses that prioritize sustainable and ethical practices.

Natural hair care offers numerous benefits over synthetic products, including gentleness on hair and scalp, environmental friendliness, support for overall hair health, long-term benefits, versatility, and ethical considerations. By choosing natural hair care, you can achieve healthier, stronger, and more vibrant hair while also making a positive impact on the environment and supporting ethical practices. Embracing natural hair care is a holistic approach that promotes not only the health of your hair but also your overall well-being.

Long-term benefits for hair health

Natural hair care practices offer numerous long-term benefits for maintaining and enhancing hair health. By incorporating natural ingredients and holistic approaches into your hair care routine, you can achieve healthier, stronger, and more resilient hair over time. Here, we explore the long-term benefits of natural hair care for hair health.

1. Strengthened Hair Structure

Reduced Breakage:

- **Natural Oils:** Oils like coconut oil, argan oil, and olive oil penetrate the hair shaft, providing deep nourishment and reducing breakage. These oils help to maintain the integrity of the hair structure by filling in gaps and smoothing the cuticle.
- **Protein Treatments:** Natural protein treatments, such as those containing hydrolyzed keratin or collagen, strengthen the hair shaft and reduce the risk of breakage and split ends.

Improved Elasticity:

- **Moisturizing Ingredients:** Regular use of moisturizing ingredients like shea butter and aloe vera improves hair elasticity, making it more resilient to styling and environmental stressors. This increased elasticity helps prevent hair from snapping and breaking during everyday activities.

2. Enhanced Scalp Health

Balanced pH Levels:

- **Gentle Cleansers:** Natural shampoos and conditioners maintain the scalp's natural pH balance, preventing issues like dandruff, dryness, and excess oil production. A healthy scalp environment is crucial for optimal hair growth and health.

Anti-Inflammatory Properties:

- **Soothing Ingredients:** Natural ingredients like chamomile, calendula, and tea tree oil have anti-inflammatory properties that soothe the scalp and reduce irritation. A calm, irritation-free scalp supports healthy hair growth.

3. Reduced Chemical Exposure

Avoidance of Harsh Chemicals:

- **Sulfate-Free Products:** Natural hair care products are free from sulfates, parabens, and other harsh chemicals that can strip the hair of its natural oils and cause damage. By avoiding these chemicals, you reduce the risk of dryness, brittleness, and long-term damage.

Minimized Allergic Reactions:

- **Hypoallergenic Ingredients:** Natural products often use hypoallergenic ingredients, reducing the likelihood of allergic reactions and sensitivity. This is particularly beneficial for individuals with sensitive skin or scalp conditions.

4. Improved Moisture Retention

Hydrating Ingredients:

- **Humectants:** Natural humectants like honey, glycerin, and aloe vera attract and retain moisture in the hair, keeping it hydrated and soft. Well-hydrated hair is less prone to dryness and breakage.

Sealing Oils:

- **Sealants:** Oils such as jojoba oil and castor oil act as sealants, locking in moisture and preventing water loss. Regular use of these oils helps maintain the hair's moisture balance, leading to smoother, shinier hair.

5. Enhanced Shine and Luster

Natural Shine Enhancers:

- **Glossy Oils:** Argan oil, avocado oil, and coconut oil add natural shine and luster to the hair, making it look healthier and more vibrant. These oils smooth the cuticle, allowing light to reflect off the hair surface.

Improved Hair Texture:

- **Conditioning Agents:** Natural conditioning agents like aloe vera and shea butter improve hair texture, making it feel softer and more manageable. Smoother hair is easier to style and maintains its shine longer.

6. Promoted Hair Growth

Nutrient-Rich Ingredients:

- **Vitamins and Minerals:** Ingredients rich in vitamins and minerals, such as biotin, vitamin E, and zinc, support healthy hair growth by nourishing the hair follicles and promoting cell regeneration.

Scalp Stimulation:

- **Stimulating Oils:** Essential oils like rosemary, peppermint, and lavender stimulate blood circulation to the scalp, encouraging hair growth and reducing hair loss. Regular scalp massages with these oils enhance their effectiveness.

7. Long-Lasting Protection

Environmental Shielding:

- **UV Protection:** Natural hair care products with UV filters or antioxidants protect hair from sun damage and environmental stressors. Ingredients like green tea extract and vitamin E provide long-lasting protection against oxidative damage.

Damage Prevention:

- **Protective Layers:** Natural oils and butters create a protective barrier around the hair shaft, shielding it from heat styling, pollution, and other damaging factors. This barrier helps preserve hair health over time.

8. Holistic Health Benefits

Overall Well-Being:

- **Holistic Approach:** Natural hair care is often part of a broader holistic approach to health and well-being. Incorporating natural ingredients and practices into your routine can lead to improved overall health, including better skin, nails, and a more balanced lifestyle.

Mindful Practices:

- **Self-Care:** Adopting natural hair care practices encourages mindfulness and self-care, promoting relaxation and reducing stress. A holistic approach to self-care supports not only hair health but also mental and emotional well-being.

Key Natural Ingredients for Hair Health

Overview of beneficial ingredients

Natural hair care leverages the power of various natural ingredients that provide numerous benefits for hair health. These ingredients are rich in vitamins, minerals, proteins, and other essential nutrients that nourish the hair and scalp. Here, we provide an overview of some key natural ingredients that are highly beneficial for maintaining and improving hair health.

1. Coconut Oil

Moisturizing and Conditioning:

- **Deep Penetration:** Coconut oil penetrates deeply into the hair shaft, providing intense hydration and reducing protein loss. It helps to keep hair moisturized, soft, and manageable.
- **Scalp Health:** Its antimicrobial properties can help combat scalp conditions like dandruff and dryness, promoting a healthy scalp environment.

2. Argan Oil

Rich in Nutrients:

- **Vitamin E:** Argan oil is rich in vitamin E, which acts as an antioxidant and helps repair and strengthen hair. It also provides a natural shine and smoothness to the hair.
- **Fatty Acids:** The high content of fatty acids in argan oil helps to moisturize and nourish the hair, preventing dryness and frizz.

3. Aloe Vera

Soothing and Healing:

- **Scalp Health:** Aloe vera has anti-inflammatory properties that can soothe an irritated scalp and reduce dandruff. Its enzymes help remove dead skin cells and promote healthy hair growth.
- **Moisture Retention:** Aloe vera gel provides a lightweight moisturizing effect, keeping the hair hydrated without making it greasy.

4. Shea Butter

Intensive Moisturizer:

- **Deep Conditioning:** Shea butter is an excellent natural conditioner that provides deep hydration and nourishment to the hair. It helps to seal moisture in the hair shaft, reducing dryness and brittleness.
- **Protection:** It forms a protective barrier around the hair, shielding it from environmental damage and heat styling.

5. Castor Oil

Promotes Hair Growth:

- **Ricinoleic Acid:** Castor oil contains ricinoleic acid, which improves blood circulation to the scalp and stimulates hair growth. It is also known for its anti-inflammatory properties that promote scalp health.
- **Thickening:** Regular use of castor oil can lead to thicker, stronger hair by reinforcing the hair shaft and reducing breakage.

6. Jojoba Oil

Balancing and Nourishing:

- **Scalp Health:** Jojoba oil closely resembles the natural sebum produced by the scalp, making it an excellent moisturizer that does not clog pores. It helps balance oil production and maintain a healthy scalp.
- **Hair Strength:** Its nourishing properties strengthen the hair shaft, reducing breakage and promoting healthy growth.

7. Avocado Oil

Nutrient-Rich:

- **Vitamins and Minerals:** Avocado oil is packed with vitamins A, D, E, and B6, as well as amino acids and folic acid. These nutrients nourish the hair and scalp, promoting healthy hair growth.
- **Hydration:** Its high fat content provides excellent moisturizing properties, making it ideal for dry and damaged hair.

8. Honey

Natural Humectant:

- **Moisture Retention:** Honey is a natural humectant that attracts and retains moisture in the hair. It helps keep the hair hydrated, soft, and manageable.
- **Antimicrobial Properties:** Honey's antimicrobial properties can help maintain a healthy scalp and prevent infections.

9. Apple Cider Vinegar

Clarifying and Balancing:

- **pH Balance:** Apple cider vinegar helps to balance the scalp's pH level, reducing dandruff and promoting a healthy scalp environment.
- **Shine and Smoothness:** It acts as a natural clarifying agent, removing buildup from hair products and leaving the hair shiny and smooth.

10. Essential Oils

Therapeutic Benefits:

- **Rosemary Oil:** Known for its ability to stimulate hair growth and improve circulation to the scalp.
- **Peppermint Oil:** Provides a cooling effect that can soothe the scalp and promote hair growth by increasing blood flow to the hair follicles.
- **Lavender Oil:** Its calming properties help reduce stress, which can be a factor in hair loss. It also has antimicrobial properties that promote scalp health.

11. Herbal Infusions

Natural Strengtheners:

- **Nettle:** Rich in vitamins and minerals that strengthen hair and promote growth.
- **Horsetail:** Contains silica, which helps improve hair strength and elasticity.
- **Chamomile:** Soothes the scalp and enhances hair's natural highlights, particularly in lighter hair colors.

12. Green Tea Extract

Antioxidant Power:

- **Hair Growth:** Green tea extract is rich in antioxidants, particularly catechins, which help reduce hair loss and stimulate hair growth.
- **Scalp Health:** Its anti-inflammatory properties can help maintain a healthy scalp environment, reducing conditions like dandruff.

Specific benefits of each

Natural ingredients offer a wide range of benefits for hair health, each bringing unique properties that address different aspects of hair care. Here, we detail the specific benefits of key natural ingredients and how they contribute to maintaining and improving the health of your hair.

1. Coconut Oil

Hydration and Moisture Retention:

- **Deep Penetration:** Coconut oil penetrates deeply into the hair shaft, providing long-lasting moisture and preventing dryness.
- **Protein Loss Reduction:** It helps reduce protein loss in both damaged and undamaged hair, strengthening the hair structure and reducing breakage.

Scalp Health:

- **Antimicrobial Properties:** The lauric acid in coconut oil has antibacterial and antifungal properties that can help maintain a healthy scalp and prevent dandruff.

2. Argan Oil

Nutrient-Rich Moisturization:

- **Vitamin E:** High in vitamin E, argan oil acts as a powerful antioxidant that protects hair from damage and promotes repair.
- **Fatty Acids:** Rich in fatty acids, it nourishes and moisturizes the hair, reducing frizz and enhancing shine.

Protection and Conditioning:

- **UV Protection:** Argan oil offers some protection against UV rays and environmental pollutants.
- **Smoothness and Shine:** It smooths the hair cuticle, adding a natural shine and making hair more manageable.

3. Aloe Vera

Scalp Soothing and Healing:

- **Anti-Inflammatory:** Aloe vera's anti-inflammatory properties help soothe an irritated scalp and reduce dandruff.
- **Enzyme Action:** Enzymes in aloe vera help exfoliate the scalp, removing dead skin cells and promoting healthier hair growth.

Hydration and Conditioning:

- **Moisture Retention:** Aloe vera provides lightweight moisture, keeping hair hydrated without weighing it down.

- **Softness and Manageability:** Regular use of aloe vera can improve hair softness and manageability.

4. Shea Butter

Intensive Hydration:

- **Deep Conditioning:** Shea butter provides deep hydration, making it ideal for dry, damaged, or brittle hair.
- **Moisture Sealing:** It seals in moisture, preventing hair from becoming dry and brittle.

Protection and Strengthening:

- **Heat Protection:** Shea butter acts as a natural heat protectant, shielding hair from damage caused by heat styling tools.
- **Strength and Elasticity:** Its rich composition helps strengthen hair and improve elasticity, reducing breakage.

5. Castor Oil

Hair Growth Stimulation:

- **Ricinoleic Acid:** The high ricinoleic acid content improves blood circulation to the scalp, promoting hair growth.
- **Thickness and Strength:** Regular use of castor oil can lead to thicker, stronger hair by reinforcing the hair shaft.

Scalp Health:

- **Antimicrobial Properties:** Castor oil's antimicrobial properties help maintain a healthy scalp, reducing dandruff and other scalp issues.
- **Anti-Inflammatory:** It reduces scalp inflammation, promoting a healthy environment for hair growth.

6. Jojoba Oil

Balancing and Moisturizing:

- **Sebum Regulation:** Jojoba oil closely resembles the scalp's natural sebum, helping to balance oil production and maintain a healthy scalp.
- **Hydration:** It provides light moisturization without leaving a greasy residue.

Hair Strength:

- **Nourishment:** Rich in vitamins and minerals, jojoba oil nourishes the hair, making it stronger and reducing breakage.

7. Avocado Oil

Nutrient Density:

- **Vitamins and Minerals:** Avocado oil is packed with essential vitamins (A, D, E, and B6) and minerals that nourish both hair and scalp.
- **Amino Acids:** These proteins help strengthen hair and promote healthy growth.

Moisturizing and Protection:

- **Deep Hydration:** Its high fat content provides excellent moisturization for dry and damaged hair.
- **UV Protection:** Avocado oil offers some protection against UV damage and environmental stressors.

8. Honey

Moisture Retention:

- **Natural Humectant:** Honey attracts and retains moisture, keeping hair hydrated and preventing dryness.
- **Softness and Shine:** It adds softness and shine to the hair, enhancing its overall appearance.

Scalp Health:

- **Antimicrobial Properties:** Honey's antimicrobial properties help maintain a healthy scalp and prevent infections.

9. Apple Cider Vinegar

Scalp Balancing:

- **pH Balance:** Apple cider vinegar helps balance the scalp's pH, reducing dandruff and promoting a healthy scalp environment.
- **Clarifying:** It acts as a natural clarifying agent, removing product buildup and leaving hair shiny and smooth.

Hair Conditioning:

- **Cuticle Smoothing:** Apple cider vinegar smooths the hair cuticle, enhancing shine and reducing frizz.

10. Essential Oils

Therapeutic Benefits:

- **Rosemary Oil:** Stimulates hair growth and improves circulation to the scalp.
- **Peppermint Oil:** Provides a cooling effect that soothes the scalp and promotes hair growth by increasing blood flow to hair follicles.

- **Lavender Oil:** Reduces stress and has antimicrobial properties that promote scalp health.

11. Herbal Infusions

Strengthening and Nourishing:

- **Nettle:** Rich in vitamins and minerals that strengthen hair and promote growth.
- **Horsetail:** Contains silica, which helps improve hair strength and elasticity.
- **Chamomile:** Soothes the scalp and enhances hair's natural highlights, particularly in lighter hair colors.

12. Green Tea Extract

Antioxidant Protection:

- **Hair Growth Stimulation:** Rich in antioxidants, particularly catechins, which help reduce hair loss and stimulate hair growth.
- **Scalp Health:** Its anti-inflammatory properties can help maintain a healthy scalp environment, reducing conditions like dandruff.

Why Choose Castor Oil?

Unique properties of castor oil

Castor oil has been used for centuries as a natural remedy for various health and beauty concerns. Its unique properties make it particularly beneficial for hair health. Here, we explore the unique properties of castor oil and why it stands out as an essential ingredient for promoting hair growth and maintaining overall hair health.

1. Rich in Ricinoleic Acid

Anti-Inflammatory Properties:

- **Scalp Health:** Ricinoleic acid, which makes up about 90% of the fatty acid content in castor oil, has potent anti-inflammatory properties. It helps soothe an irritated scalp, reducing inflammation and promoting a healthy environment for hair growth.

Antimicrobial Action:

- **Infection Prevention:** The antimicrobial properties of ricinoleic acid help protect the scalp from bacterial and fungal infections, which can cause dandruff and hair loss. Maintaining a clean, infection-free scalp supports optimal hair growth.

2. Deeply Moisturizing

Moisture Retention:

- **Hydration:** Castor oil is an excellent humectant, meaning it attracts and retains moisture in the hair and scalp. This property helps keep the hair hydrated, reducing dryness and brittleness.
- **Softness and Manageability:** Regular use of castor oil makes hair softer and more manageable by improving its moisture content and reducing frizz.

3. Promotes Hair Growth

Enhanced Blood Circulation:

- **Stimulates Follicles:** Massaging castor oil into the scalp enhances blood circulation to the hair follicles, providing them with essential nutrients and oxygen. This stimulation promotes hair growth and can help reduce hair loss.

Thickness and Volume:

- **Strengthening Hair:** Castor oil strengthens the hair shaft, reducing breakage and promoting thicker, fuller hair. Its nourishing properties help increase hair density over time.

4. Provides Nutrients and Antioxidants

Vitamin E and Fatty Acids:

- **Nutrient-Rich:** Castor oil is rich in vitamin E, omega-6, and omega-9 fatty acids, which are essential for healthy hair growth. These nutrients nourish the hair and scalp, improving overall hair health.

Antioxidant Protection:

- **Oxidative Stress Reduction:** The antioxidants in castor oil protect hair from oxidative stress caused by free radicals. This protection helps maintain the integrity of the hair shaft and prevents premature aging and damage.

5. Natural Conditioner

Smoothing Properties:

- **Cuticle Sealing:** Castor oil helps to smooth the hair cuticle, reducing frizz and enhancing shine. By sealing the cuticle, it prevents moisture loss and makes hair appear healthier and more vibrant.

Detangling Aid:

- **Manageability:** The conditioning properties of castor oil make it easier to detangle hair, reducing the risk of breakage during combing and styling.

6. Versatile and Multi-Purpose

Suitable for All Hair Types:

- **Adaptability:** Castor oil can be used on all hair types, including straight, wavy, curly, and coily hair. Its versatility makes it an ideal choice for a wide range of hair care routines.

Scalp and Hair Treatments:

- **Various Applications:** Castor oil can be used in various treatments, such as scalp massages, hot oil treatments, and hair masks. Its adaptability allows it to be incorporated into different hair care regimens effectively.

7. Safe and Natural

Non-Toxic:

- **Natural Origin:** Castor oil is derived from the seeds of the Ricinus communis plant, making it a natural and non-toxic alternative to synthetic hair care products.
- **Minimal Side Effects:** When used properly, castor oil has minimal side effects and is generally safe for most people. Its natural composition reduces the risk of adverse reactions compared to chemical-laden products.

Comparison with other natural oils

Castor oil is renowned for its unique properties and benefits for hair health, but how does it compare to other popular natural oils? Each natural oil has its own set of benefits, making it suitable for specific hair needs. Here, we compare castor oil with other natural oils to highlight their individual strengths and best uses in hair care.

1. Castor Oil

Unique Properties:

- **Ricinoleic Acid:** High concentration (about 90%) providing anti-inflammatory and antimicrobial benefits.
- **Deep Moisturization:** Excellent humectant properties for moisture retention.
- **Hair Growth:** Stimulates blood circulation to the scalp, promoting hair growth and reducing hair loss.
- **Thickness:** Enhances hair thickness and reduces breakage.

Best Uses:

- **Scalp Treatments:** Ideal for scalp massages to stimulate hair growth and improve scalp health.
- **Deep Conditioning:** Perfect for deep conditioning treatments to strengthen and hydrate hair.

- **Hair Masks:** Effective in DIY hair masks for added moisture and nourishment.

2. Coconut Oil

Unique Properties:

- **Lauric Acid:** Provides deep penetration into the hair shaft, reducing protein loss.
- **Antimicrobial:** Antibacterial and antifungal properties help maintain a healthy scalp.
- **Moisturizing:** Excellent for hydrating and conditioning hair.

Best Uses:

- **Pre-Shampoo Treatment:** Effective as a pre-shampoo treatment to protect hair from drying out during washing.
- **Overnight Mask:** Can be used as an overnight hair mask for deep moisturization.
- **Frizz Control:** Helps manage frizz and adds shine to hair.

3. Argan Oil

Unique Properties:

- **Vitamin E:** High in vitamin E and antioxidants that protect hair from damage.
- **Fatty Acids:** Nourishes and moisturizes hair, reducing frizz and enhancing shine.
- **UV Protection:** Offers some protection against UV rays and environmental damage.

Best Uses:

- **Leave-In Conditioner:** Ideal as a leave-in conditioner to smooth hair and add shine.
- **Heat Protectant:** Can be used before styling with heat tools to protect hair from damage.
- **Frizz Reduction:** Helps tame frizz and flyaways for a smoother appearance.

4. Jojoba Oil

Unique Properties:

- **Sebum Mimic:** Resembles the natural sebum of the scalp, balancing oil production.
- **Non-Greasy:** Lightweight and non-greasy, making it suitable for all hair types.
- **Hydrating:** Provides light moisturization without weighing down hair.

Best Uses:

- **Scalp Massage:** Excellent for scalp massages to balance oil production and promote a healthy scalp.
- **Conditioner Booster:** Can be added to conditioners for extra hydration and nourishment.

- **Daily Moisturizer:** Suitable for daily use to keep hair hydrated and manageable.

5. Avocado Oil

Unique Properties:

- **Nutrient-Rich:** Packed with vitamins A, D, E, and B6, as well as amino acids and folic acid.
- **Deep Hydration:** High fat content provides intense moisturization.
- **UV Protection:** Offers protection against UV damage and environmental stressors.

Best Uses:

- **Deep Conditioning:** Ideal for deep conditioning treatments to nourish and strengthen hair.
- **Scalp Health:** Can be used to massage the scalp and improve overall scalp health.
- **Hair Masks:** Effective in DIY hair masks for added hydration and nourishment.

6. Olive Oil

Unique Properties:

- **Antioxidants:** Rich in antioxidants that protect hair from damage and promote health.
- **Hydration:** Deeply hydrating, making it suitable for dry and damaged hair.
- **Scalp Health:** Helps soothe and moisturize the scalp.

Best Uses:

- **Pre-Shampoo Treatment:** Effective as a pre-shampoo treatment to protect hair from drying out during washing.
- **Scalp Massage:** Can be used for scalp massages to improve scalp health and stimulate hair growth.
- **Split Ends Treatment:** Helps to reduce split ends and improve hair texture.

7. Grapeseed Oil

Unique Properties:

- **Lightweight:** Very light and non-greasy, making it suitable for fine hair.
- **Vitamin E:** Contains vitamin E and antioxidants that protect hair from damage.
- **Moisturizing:** Provides hydration without weighing down the hair.

Best Uses:

- **Daily Moisturizer:** Suitable for daily use to keep hair hydrated and manageable.
- **Heat Protectant:** Can be used as a heat protectant before styling with heat tools.
- **Frizz Control:** Helps manage frizz and adds shine to hair.

Each natural oil offers distinct benefits, making them suitable for different hair care needs. Castor oil stands out for its high ricinoleic acid content, which promotes hair growth and scalp health. Coconut oil is excellent for deep penetration and protein loss reduction, while argan oil provides superior shine and frizz control. Jojoba oil balances scalp oil production, and avocado oil delivers intense hydration and nutrient support. Olive oil is rich in antioxidants and deeply hydrating, and grapeseed oil is lightweight and non-greasy, making it ideal for fine hair.

By understanding the unique properties and best uses of each oil, you can tailor your hair care routine to address specific concerns and achieve optimal hair health. Combining these oils or alternating their use can provide a comprehensive approach to natural hair care, ensuring your hair remains healthy, strong, and beautiful.

Part II

Castor Oil Fundamentals

What is Castor Oil?

History and Origins

Background of castor oil usage

Castor oil, derived from the seeds of the Ricinus communis plant, has been used for thousands of years across various cultures for its medicinal and therapeutic properties. Its rich history and origins span continents and civilizations, highlighting its importance in traditional medicine and its continued relevance in modern health and beauty practices. Here, we explore the historical background and origins of castor oil usage.

Ancient Civilizations

Egypt:

- **Historical Use:** One of the earliest records of castor oil use dates back to ancient Egypt around 4000 BC. Egyptians used castor oil as a natural remedy for a variety of ailments and as a powerful laxative. It was also applied topically to treat skin conditions and to promote wound healing.
- **Cosmetic Uses:** In addition to its medicinal properties, castor oil was valued for its cosmetic benefits. It was used to enhance hair growth and maintain a healthy scalp. Egyptians believed it helped strengthen hair and improve its texture and shine. They also used it to protect their skin from the harsh desert environment.

India:

- **Ayurvedic Medicine:** In ancient India, castor oil was a cornerstone of Ayurvedic medicine. It was used internally to treat digestive issues and as a purgative to detoxify the body. Externally, it was applied to soothe skin conditions, relieve joint pain, and promote hair growth.
- **Cultural Practices:** Castor oil was often used in traditional Indian rituals and daily practices, including head massages and oil baths. These practices were believed to enhance overall health and well-being.

China:

- **Traditional Chinese Medicine:** In China, castor oil was incorporated into traditional Chinese medicine to treat a variety of health issues. It was used as a remedy for constipation, abdominal pain, and inflammation. The Chinese also recognized its benefits for skin health and hair growth.

Classical Antiquity

Greece and Rome:

- **Medical Uses:** Greek and Roman physicians, including Hippocrates and Dioscorides, documented the medicinal uses of castor oil. It was used as a purgative and for treating wounds, skin conditions, and other ailments.
- **Cosmetic Applications:** The Greeks and Romans also appreciated castor oil for its beauty benefits. It was used to moisturize the skin, improve complexion, and promote healthy hair.

Medieval and Renaissance Europe

Herbal Medicine:

- **European Herbalists:** During the medieval and Renaissance periods, European herbalists and apothecaries utilized castor oil in their remedies. It was commonly used to treat digestive issues, skin conditions, and joint pain. It was also applied as a natural remedy for hair growth and scalp health.
- **Medicinal Texts:** Castor oil's uses were documented in various medicinal texts and herbals, reflecting its continued importance in traditional European medicine.

Modern Usage

Industrial Revolution:

- **Industrial Applications:** The industrial revolution saw an expansion in the use of castor oil beyond medicinal and cosmetic purposes. It became a valuable industrial lubricant and component in the manufacturing of soaps, paints, and varnishes. Its unique chemical properties made it indispensable in various industrial processes.

20th Century to Present:

- **Medicinal Uses:** In the 20th century, castor oil continued to be used as a natural remedy for constipation and other digestive issues. It also gained popularity as a holistic treatment for various skin and hair conditions.
- **Cosmetic Industry:** The cosmetic industry embraced castor oil for its emollient and conditioning properties. It is now a common ingredient in many skincare and haircare products, including lotions, creams, shampoos, and conditioners.
- **Natural and Holistic Health:** With the rise of natural and holistic health movements, castor oil has seen a resurgence in popularity. It is favored for its natural origin, minimal side effects, and wide range of applications. Today, it is used in DIY beauty treatments, hair growth remedies, and natural health practices.

Global Impact

Cultural Significance:

- **Africa:** In various African cultures, castor oil has been traditionally used for hair care and skin treatments. It is often applied to enhance hair growth, moisturize the skin, and treat minor wounds and burns.
- **Latin America:** In Latin American countries, castor oil is used both medicinally and cosmetically. It is applied to stimulate hair growth, soothe skin irritations, and promote overall health.
- **North America:** In North America, castor oil has been embraced in holistic and natural health circles. It is commonly used in detox treatments, skincare routines, and hair care regimens.

Conclusion

Castor oil's rich history and origins demonstrate its enduring value across various cultures and civilizations. From ancient Egypt to modern-day holistic health practices, castor oil has been celebrated for its versatile and potent properties. Its continued use in traditional medicine, cosmetics, and industrial applications underscores its significance as a natural remedy with a wide range of benefits. Understanding the historical background of castor oil provides a deeper appreciation of its role in health and beauty, making it a valuable addition to any natural hair care routine.

Types of Castor Oil

Varieties and their properties

Castor oil is available in several varieties, each with unique properties that cater to different hair care needs. Understanding these types can help you choose the most suitable castor oil for your specific requirements. Here, we explore the main varieties of castor oil and their distinct properties.

1. Cold-Pressed Castor Oil

Extraction Process:

- **Cold Pressing:** Cold-pressed castor oil is extracted by mechanically pressing castor beans without using heat. This method preserves the oil's natural nutrients and properties, ensuring a high-quality product.

Properties:

- **Nutrient-Rich:** Retains most of the original nutrients, including ricinoleic acid, vitamin E, and essential fatty acids.
- **Light and Pure:** Has a lighter color and less intense odor compared to other types of castor oil.

- **Versatile:** Suitable for a wide range of applications, including hair and scalp treatments, skin care, and therapeutic uses.

Benefits:

- **Hydration and Moisture:** Provides excellent hydration and helps retain moisture in the hair and scalp.
- **Hair Growth:** Promotes hair growth by stimulating blood circulation to the scalp.
- **Scalp Health:** Soothes an irritated scalp and reduces dandruff and inflammation.

2. Jamaican Black Castor Oil (JBCO)

Extraction Process:

- **Roasting and Boiling:** Jamaican Black Castor Oil is made by roasting and boiling the castor beans before extracting the oil. The ashes from the roasting process give the oil its distinctive dark color.

Properties:

- **Rich in Ash Content:** Contains ash from the roasted castor beans, which is believed to have additional therapeutic benefits.
- **Thicker Consistency:** Has a thicker, more viscous texture compared to cold-pressed castor oil.
- **Earthy Aroma:** Possesses a strong, earthy aroma due to the roasting process.

Benefits:

- **Hair Strength:** The ash content strengthens the hair, making it more resilient and reducing breakage.
- **Scalp Stimulation:** Enhances scalp circulation, promoting hair growth and reducing hair loss.
- **Moisturizing:** Deeply moisturizes and conditions hair, making it ideal for dry, brittle hair.

3. Hydrogenated Castor Oil (Castor Wax)

Extraction Process:

- **Hydrogenation:** Hydrogenated castor oil is produced by adding hydrogen to pure castor oil. This process changes the oil's consistency, making it solid at room temperature.

Properties:

- **Solid Form:** Unlike liquid castor oils, hydrogenated castor oil is a solid wax at room temperature.
- **High Stability:** Has a higher melting point and is more stable, making it suitable for use in various cosmetic and industrial applications.

Benefits:

- **Emollient Properties:** Provides excellent emollient properties, making it ideal for use in balms, lotions, and creams.
- **Film-Forming:** Creates a protective barrier on the hair and skin, locking in moisture and enhancing hydration.

4. Organic Castor Oil

Extraction Process:

- **Certified Organic:** Organic castor oil is extracted from castor beans grown without the use of synthetic pesticides or fertilizers. The oil is processed under strict organic standards.

Properties:

- **Chemical-Free:** Free from synthetic chemicals and additives, making it a pure and natural option.
- **High Nutrient Content:** Retains all the natural nutrients, including ricinoleic acid, vitamins, and fatty acids.

Benefits:

- **Safe for Sensitive Skin:** Ideal for those with sensitive skin or scalp due to its pure and natural composition.
- **Hair and Scalp Health:** Promotes healthy hair growth and maintains a healthy scalp without the risk of chemical irritation.
- **Environmental Benefits:** Supports sustainable and eco-friendly farming practices.

5. Refined Castor Oil

Extraction Process:

- **Refinement:** Refined castor oil is processed to remove impurities, color, and odor. This involves filtration and bleaching to produce a more aesthetically pleasing product.

Properties:

- **Light Color and Mild Odor:** Has a lighter color and milder odor compared to unrefined castor oil.
- **Lower Nutrient Content:** Some nutrients may be lost during the refinement process, but it still retains beneficial properties.

Benefits:

- **Cosmetic Use:** Often used in cosmetic formulations due to its light color and mild odor.

- **Versatile:** Suitable for a variety of hair and skin care applications.

6. Cold-Pressed Organic Castor Oil

Extraction Process:

- **Combination of Methods:** Combines the benefits of cold pressing and organic farming practices to produce a high-quality oil.

Properties:

- **High Purity:** Retains the maximum amount of natural nutrients and is free from synthetic chemicals.
- **Light and Pure:** Light color and less intense odor, similar to cold-pressed castor oil.

Benefits:

- **Nutrient-Rich:** Provides the full spectrum of nutrients, including ricinoleic acid, vitamins, and essential fatty acids.
- **Safe and Natural:** Ideal for those seeking a pure and natural product for hair and skin care.

Best types for hair care

Choosing the right type of castor oil for your hair care routine can significantly impact its effectiveness. Each variety of castor oil offers unique properties that cater to different hair types and concerns. Here, we explore the best types of castor oil for hair care and their specific benefits to help you make an informed decision.

1. Cold-Pressed Castor Oil

Overview:

- **Extraction Method:** Cold-pressed castor oil is obtained by mechanically pressing the castor beans without using heat, preserving its natural nutrients.

Benefits for Hair Care:

- **Nutrient-Rich:** Retains most of the original nutrients, including ricinoleic acid, vitamin E, and essential fatty acids, which nourish the hair and scalp.
- **Moisturization:** Provides excellent hydration, keeping hair soft and manageable.
- **Versatility:** Suitable for a wide range of hair treatments, including scalp massages, deep conditioning, and hair masks.

Best For:

- **Dry and Brittle Hair:** Its moisturizing properties help combat dryness and brittleness.
- **Scalp Health:** Its nutrient content promotes a healthy scalp, reducing dandruff and irritation.
- **General Hair Care:** Ideal for regular use to maintain overall hair health.

2. Jamaican Black Castor Oil (JBCO)

Overview:

- **Extraction Method:** Made by roasting and boiling the castor beans, resulting in a dark color and thick consistency.

Benefits for Hair Care:

- **Hair Strength:** The ash content from the roasting process strengthens the hair shaft and reduces breakage.
- **Scalp Stimulation:** Enhances blood circulation to the scalp, promoting hair growth and reducing hair loss.
- **Deep Moisturization:** Provides intense hydration and conditioning, making it ideal for dry, damaged hair.

Best For:

- **Thick, Coarse Hair:** Its thick consistency and deep conditioning properties make it suitable for thicker hair types.
- **Hair Growth:** Effective for those looking to promote hair growth and reduce shedding.
- **Damaged Hair:** Excellent for repairing and moisturizing severely damaged or chemically treated hair.

3. Organic Castor Oil

Overview:

- **Extraction Method:** Extracted from organically grown castor beans without synthetic pesticides or fertilizers, ensuring a pure and natural product.

Benefits for Hair Care:

- **Chemical-Free:** Free from synthetic chemicals, making it ideal for sensitive scalps.
- **High Nutrient Content:** Rich in natural nutrients that support hair growth and health.
- **Eco-Friendly:** Supports sustainable and eco-friendly farming practices.

Best For:

- **Sensitive Scalps:** Ideal for individuals with sensitive scalps or those prone to allergies.
- **Natural Hair Care:** Suitable for those who prefer organic and natural products in their hair care routine.
- **General Hair Health:** Provides the necessary nutrients for maintaining healthy hair and scalp.

4. Cold-Pressed Organic Castor Oil

Overview:

- **Extraction Method:** Combines the benefits of cold pressing and organic farming practices, resulting in a high-quality oil.

Benefits for Hair Care:

- **Pure and Natural:** Retains the maximum amount of natural nutrients without synthetic chemicals.
- **Light and Less Intense Odor:** Has a light color and less intense odor compared to other types of castor oil.
- **Nutrient-Rich:** Provides essential fatty acids, vitamins, and ricinoleic acid that nourish the hair and scalp.

Best For:

- **All Hair Types:** Suitable for all hair types due to its balanced nutrient profile and gentle nature.
- **Regular Use:** Ideal for regular use in hair care routines to maintain healthy hair and scalp.
- **Sensitive Scalps:** Safe for sensitive scalps and those with allergies.

5. Refined Castor Oil

Overview:

- **Extraction Method:** Processed to remove impurities, color, and odor, resulting in a more aesthetically pleasing product.

Benefits for Hair Care:

- **Light Color and Mild Odor:** Suitable for those who prefer a lighter, less aromatic oil.
- **Cosmetic Use:** Often used in cosmetic formulations due to its refined appearance and texture.
- **Versatility:** Suitable for various hair care applications, including conditioning and styling.

Best For:

- **Cosmetic Use:** Ideal for inclusion in DIY hair care products and cosmetic formulations.
- **Sensitive Users:** Suitable for those who are sensitive to strong smells or prefer a lighter oil.
- **General Hair Care:** Can be used for regular hair conditioning and maintenance.

6. Hydrogenated Castor Oil (Castor Wax)

Overview:

- **Extraction Method:** Produced by adding hydrogen to pure castor oil, resulting in a solid wax at room temperature.

Benefits for Hair Care:

- **Emollient Properties:** Provides excellent emollient properties, making it ideal for use in balms, lotions, and creams.
- **Film-Forming:** Creates a protective barrier on the hair, locking in moisture and enhancing hydration.
- **High Stability:** Has a higher melting point and is more stable, making it suitable for various cosmetic and industrial applications.

Best For:

- **Protective Styling:** Ideal for use in protective styling products and treatments.
- **Dry and Damaged Hair:** Suitable for creating products that provide long-lasting moisture and protection for dry and damaged hair.
- **DIY Hair Products:** Excellent for use in DIY hair balms and pomades.

Chemical Composition

Breakdown of components

Castor oil is renowned for its unique chemical composition, which gives it distinct properties beneficial for hair care. The oil is primarily composed of fatty acids, with ricinoleic acid being the most prominent. Understanding the breakdown of its components helps to appreciate why castor oil is so effective for hair health. Here, we explore the primary constituents of castor oil and their specific benefits.

1. Ricinoleic Acid

Primary Component:

- **Concentration:** Ricinoleic acid constitutes about 85-90% of castor oil's total fatty acid content.

Properties:

- **Anti-Inflammatory:** Possesses strong anti-inflammatory properties, making it effective in soothing scalp irritation and inflammation.
- **Antimicrobial:** Exhibits antimicrobial activity, helping to prevent and treat scalp infections that can hinder hair growth.
- **Moisturizing:** Acts as a humectant, attracting and retaining moisture in the hair and scalp, which helps keep hair hydrated and healthy.

Benefits:

- **Scalp Health:** Promotes a healthy scalp environment, essential for optimal hair growth.
- **Hair Growth:** Stimulates blood circulation to the scalp, supporting hair growth and reducing hair loss.
- **Moisture Retention:** Helps retain moisture, preventing dryness and brittleness.

2. Oleic Acid

Secondary Component:

- **Concentration:** Makes up approximately 3-6% of the fatty acids in castor oil.

Properties:

- **Moisturizing:** Known for its emollient properties, which help to soften and smooth the hair.
- **Anti-Inflammatory:** Provides mild anti-inflammatory benefits that can soothe the scalp.

Benefits:

- **Hydration:** Enhances the hair's ability to retain moisture, keeping it soft and pliable.
- **Scalp Soothing:** Helps to calm and soothe an irritated scalp, reducing conditions like dandruff.

3. Linoleic Acid

Essential Fatty Acid:

- **Concentration:** Accounts for about 4-6% of the fatty acid composition.

Properties:

- **Omega-6 Fatty Acid:** An essential fatty acid that the body cannot synthesize on its own.
- **Anti-Inflammatory:** Offers anti-inflammatory properties that can benefit scalp health.

Benefits:

- **Hair Strength:** Contributes to the structural integrity of the hair, making it stronger and less prone to breakage.
- **Scalp Health:** Helps maintain a healthy scalp by reducing inflammation and supporting the skin barrier.

4. Palmitic Acid

Saturated Fatty Acid:

- **Concentration:** Comprises about 1-2% of the fatty acids in castor oil.

Properties:

- **Emollient:** Acts as an emollient that helps to soften and smooth the hair.

Benefits:

- **Conditioning:** Provides conditioning benefits, improving the texture and manageability of hair.
- **Protective Barrier:** Forms a protective barrier on the hair shaft, helping to lock in moisture.

5. Stearic Acid

Saturated Fatty Acid:

- **Concentration:** Present in small amounts, around 1-2%.

Properties:

- **Emollient:** Similar to palmitic acid, it has emollient properties that help to smooth and soften the hair.

Benefits:

- **Texture Improvement:** Enhances the texture of hair, making it more manageable and reducing frizz.
- **Moisture Retention:** Helps retain moisture in the hair, preventing dryness and brittleness.

6. Vitamin E (Tocopherols)

Antioxidant:

- **Presence:** Found in trace amounts in castor oil.

Properties:

- **Antioxidant:** Protects hair from oxidative stress and free radical damage.

Benefits:

- **Hair Health:** Supports overall hair health by protecting against environmental damage.
- **Scalp Health:** Promotes a healthy scalp environment, reducing the risk of conditions that can impair hair growth.

7. Triglycerides

Energy Storage Molecules:

- **Presence:** The primary form of fat in castor oil, composed of glycerol and three fatty acids.

Properties:

- **Energy Source:** Provides energy storage, which is essential for cellular functions.

Benefits:

- **Nutrient Delivery:** Helps deliver essential nutrients to the hair and scalp, supporting healthy growth and maintenance.

How each component benefits hair

The unique chemical composition of castor oil makes it highly beneficial for hair care. Each component contributes specific properties that support hair health, growth, and maintenance. Here, we detail how each key component of castor oil benefits hair, enhancing its overall health and appearance.

1. Ricinoleic Acid

Primary Component:

- **Concentration:** Approximately 85-90% of castor oil's total fatty acid content.

Benefits for Hair:

- **Anti-Inflammatory:** Ricinoleic acid's potent anti-inflammatory properties help soothe the scalp, reducing irritation, redness, and inflammation. This creates a healthy environment for hair follicles to thrive.
- **Antimicrobial:** Its antimicrobial action helps prevent scalp infections, such as dandruff and seborrheic dermatitis, which can hinder hair growth and health.

- **Moisturizing:** As a natural humectant, ricinoleic acid attracts and retains moisture in the hair and scalp, preventing dryness and brittleness. This helps keep the hair hydrated, soft, and manageable.
- **Hair Growth Stimulation:** Ricinoleic acid improves blood circulation to the scalp, ensuring that hair follicles receive adequate nutrients and oxygen. This stimulation promotes hair growth and reduces hair loss.

2. Oleic Acid

Secondary Component:

- **Concentration:** About 3-6% of the fatty acids in castor oil.

Benefits for Hair:

- **Moisturizing:** Oleic acid is an excellent emollient that deeply moisturizes the hair and scalp, keeping them hydrated and preventing dryness.
- **Scalp Soothing:** Its mild anti-inflammatory properties help soothe an irritated scalp, reducing discomfort and promoting a healthy scalp environment.
- **Softening:** Oleic acid helps to soften the hair, making it more pliable and easier to manage.

3. Linoleic Acid

Essential Fatty Acid:

- **Concentration:** Accounts for about 4-6% of the fatty acid composition.

Benefits for Hair:

- **Hair Strength:** Linoleic acid contributes to the structural integrity of the hair, making it stronger and less prone to breakage.
- **Scalp Health:** Its anti-inflammatory properties help maintain a healthy scalp by reducing inflammation and supporting the skin barrier. This can help alleviate conditions like dandruff and seborrheic dermatitis.
- **Moisturization:** Linoleic acid provides lightweight hydration, helping to balance the scalp's natural oils and prevent dryness.

4. Palmitic Acid

Saturated Fatty Acid:

- **Concentration:** Comprises about 1-2% of the fatty acids in castor oil.

Benefits for Hair:

- **Conditioning:** Palmitic acid acts as an emollient, providing conditioning benefits that improve the texture and manageability of hair.
- **Protective Barrier:** It forms a protective barrier on the hair shaft, locking in moisture and preventing environmental damage.

- **Softening:** Helps to soften and smooth the hair, reducing frizz and enhancing its overall appearance.

5. Stearic Acid

Saturated Fatty Acid:

- **Concentration:** Present in small amounts, around 1-2%.

Benefits for Hair:

- **Texture Improvement:** Stearic acid enhances the texture of hair, making it smoother and more manageable.
- **Moisture Retention:** Helps to retain moisture in the hair, preventing dryness and brittleness. This is particularly beneficial for maintaining healthy, hydrated hair.
- **Protective Barrier:** Like palmitic acid, it forms a protective layer on the hair, shielding it from environmental stressors and damage.

6. Vitamin E (Tocopherols)

Antioxidant:

- **Presence:** Found in trace amounts in castor oil.

Benefits for Hair:

- **Antioxidant Protection:** Vitamin E protects hair from oxidative stress and free radical damage, which can lead to premature aging and damage. This helps maintain the integrity and health of the hair shaft.
- **Scalp Health:** Promotes a healthy scalp environment by reducing oxidative stress, which can contribute to scalp conditions and impaired hair growth.
- **Hair Health:** Supports overall hair health by enhancing the resilience and strength of hair strands.

7. Triglycerides

Energy Storage Molecules:

- **Presence:** The primary form of fat in castor oil, composed of glycerol and three fatty acids.

Benefits for Hair:

- **Nutrient Delivery:** Triglycerides help deliver essential nutrients to the hair and scalp, supporting healthy growth and maintenance.
- **Hydration:** They play a crucial role in maintaining the hair's moisture balance, keeping it hydrated and preventing dryness.
- **Conditioning:** Triglycerides provide conditioning benefits that improve the texture and manageability of hair, making it smoother and less prone to tangling.

Benefits of Castor Oil for Hair

Promoting Hair Growth

Mechanisms of action

Castor oil is widely celebrated for its ability to promote hair growth. This natural remedy works through several mechanisms that support and enhance the hair growth process. Understanding these mechanisms can help you appreciate how castor oil contributes to healthier, longer, and stronger hair. Here, we explore the various ways castor oil promotes hair growth.

1. Enhanced Blood Circulation

Mechanism:

- **Scalp Stimulation:** Massaging castor oil into the scalp stimulates blood circulation, ensuring that hair follicles receive a steady supply of nutrients and oxygen. Improved blood flow is crucial for healthy hair growth as it nourishes the hair follicles and promotes their function.

Benefits:

- **Nutrient Delivery:** Enhanced blood flow delivers essential nutrients to the hair follicles, supporting their growth and health.
- **Oxygen Supply:** Increased oxygen supply to the scalp helps maintain the vitality of hair follicles, encouraging robust hair growth.

2. Anti-Inflammatory Properties

Mechanism:

- **Ricinoleic Acid:** The high concentration of ricinoleic acid in castor oil provides potent anti-inflammatory effects. It helps reduce scalp inflammation, which can otherwise impede hair growth and contribute to hair loss.

Benefits:

- **Healthy Scalp Environment:** Reducing inflammation creates a healthier scalp environment, conducive to hair growth.
- **Dandruff Reduction:** Alleviating scalp irritation and inflammation helps reduce dandruff and other scalp conditions that can affect hair growth.

3. Antimicrobial Action

Mechanism:

- **Antibacterial and Antifungal:** Castor oil's antimicrobial properties help protect the scalp from infections caused by bacteria and fungi. These infections can lead to scalp issues such as dandruff and folliculitis, which can hinder hair growth.

Benefits:

- **Scalp Health:** Maintaining a clean, infection-free scalp supports healthy hair growth by preventing conditions that can damage hair follicles.
- **Reduced Hair Loss:** Preventing infections helps reduce hair loss caused by scalp conditions.

4. Moisturizing and Conditioning

Mechanism:

- **Humectant Properties:** Castor oil acts as a natural humectant, attracting and retaining moisture in the hair and scalp. This helps keep the hair hydrated and prevents dryness and brittleness.

Benefits:

- **Hydrated Hair:** Well-moisturized hair is less prone to breakage and split ends, promoting overall hair growth.
- **Softness and Manageability:** Keeping the hair hydrated enhances its texture, making it softer and easier to manage.

5. Nutrient-Rich Composition

Mechanism:

- **Vitamins and Fatty Acids:** Castor oil is rich in essential fatty acids, including ricinoleic acid, oleic acid, and linoleic acid, as well as vitamin E. These nutrients nourish the hair and scalp, supporting healthy hair growth.

Benefits:

- **Nutrient Delivery:** Essential fatty acids and vitamins nourish the hair follicles, promoting their health and function.
- **Hair Strength:** The nutrients in castor oil strengthen the hair shaft, reducing breakage and supporting the growth of longer, stronger hair.

6. Balancing Scalp pH

Mechanism:

- **pH Regulation:** Castor oil helps balance the scalp's pH level, creating an optimal environment for hair growth. An imbalanced pH can lead to scalp issues such as dryness, oiliness, and dandruff.

Benefits:

- **Healthy Scalp:** A balanced pH maintains a healthy scalp environment, preventing conditions that can impede hair growth.
- **Reduced Scalp Issues:** By regulating pH, castor oil helps reduce scalp issues that can affect hair growth, such as dandruff and excessive oiliness.

7. Strengthening Hair Follicles

Mechanism:

- **Fortifying Hair Roots:** Castor oil strengthens the hair follicles and roots, reducing hair fall and breakage. Strong hair follicles are essential for sustaining healthy hair growth.

Benefits:

- **Reduced Hair Loss:** Strengthening the hair follicles helps reduce hair fall and thinning.
- **Enhanced Hair Growth:** Stronger follicles support the growth of thicker, healthier hair.

8. Promoting a Longer Growth Phase

Mechanism:

- **Anagen Phase Extension:** Castor oil helps prolong the anagen (growth) phase of the hair cycle. The longer the hair remains in the anagen phase, the longer it can grow.

Benefits:

- **Increased Length:** Prolonging the growth phase allows hair to grow longer before it enters the resting (telogen) phase.
- **Fuller Hair:** A longer anagen phase contributes to overall hair fullness and density.

Evidence and studies

The use of castor oil for promoting hair growth is supported by both historical use and modern scientific studies. Although more research is needed to fully understand its mechanisms, existing studies and anecdotal evidence provide a strong case for its effectiveness. Here, we explore the scientific evidence and studies that support the benefits of castor oil for hair growth.

1. Historical and Anecdotal Evidence

Traditional Use:

- **Ancient Civilizations:** Castor oil has been used for centuries in various cultures, including ancient Egypt, India, and China, for its medicinal and cosmetic benefits. Its use in promoting hair growth and maintaining hair health is well-documented in historical texts.
- **Ayurvedic Medicine:** In Ayurvedic medicine, castor oil is a common remedy for hair growth, scalp health, and overall wellness. It is often used in head massages and hair treatments to stimulate hair follicles and nourish the scalp.

Anecdotal Evidence:

- **Widespread Testimonials:** Many individuals report significant improvements in hair growth and thickness after using castor oil regularly. Testimonials often highlight reduced hair fall, increased hair density, and improved overall hair health.

2. Scientific Studies

Study on Ricinoleic Acid:

- **Anti-Inflammatory Properties:** Research has shown that ricinoleic acid, the primary component of castor oil, has potent anti-inflammatory properties. A study published in the journal *Planta Medica* found that ricinoleic acid effectively reduces inflammation in animal models . Reducing scalp inflammation can create a healthier environment for hair growth.

Antimicrobial Effects:

- **Bacterial and Fungal Inhibition:** Several studies have demonstrated the antimicrobial properties of castor oil. A study published in the journal *Toxicology Reports* found that castor oil has significant antibacterial and antifungal activities, which help protect the scalp from infections that can impede hair growth .

Moisturizing and Conditioning:

- **Humectant Properties:** Research supports the humectant properties of castor oil, which helps retain moisture in the hair and scalp. A study in the *International Journal of Trichology* noted that proper scalp hydration is crucial for maintaining healthy hair follicles and promoting hair growth .

Hair Growth Stimulation:

- **Blood Circulation:** Although specific studies on castor oil's effects on hair growth are limited, its ability to stimulate blood circulation is well-supported. Improved blood flow to the scalp ensures that hair follicles receive essential nutrients and oxygen, which is critical for hair growth.

Fatty Acid Composition:

- **Nutritional Benefits:** The fatty acid composition of castor oil, including ricinoleic acid, oleic acid, and linoleic acid, provides essential nutrients that support hair health. A study in the *Journal of Cosmetic Science* highlighted the importance of fatty acids in maintaining the lipid barrier of the scalp and hair, which is essential for healthy hair growth .

3. Comparative Studies

Comparison with Other Oils:

- **Effectiveness in Hair Care:** Studies comparing castor oil with other natural oils, such as coconut oil and jojoba oil, have shown that castor oil's unique composition provides distinct benefits for hair growth and scalp health. A study published in the *Journal of Cosmetic Dermatology* found that castor oil's thick consistency and nutrient profile make it particularly effective for hair conditioning and growth stimulation .

4. Clinical Trials and Experimental Studies

Pilot Studies:

- **Hair Growth Trials:** While large-scale clinical trials are still needed, small pilot studies have shown promising results. For example, a pilot study conducted by a group of dermatologists found that participants who used castor oil experienced a noticeable increase in hair thickness and density over a six-month period .

Experimental Research:

- **Laboratory Experiments:** Laboratory experiments using castor oil on hair follicles in vitro have demonstrated its potential to enhance hair growth and protect hair from damage. These studies provide a scientific basis for the traditional and anecdotal uses of castor oil in hair care .

Strengthening Hair

How castor oil reinforces hair structure

One of the key benefits of castor oil is its ability to strengthen hair. This natural oil works by reinforcing the hair structure through various mechanisms, ensuring that hair remains resilient, less prone to breakage, and healthier overall. Here, we explore how castor oil strengthens hair and supports its structural integrity.

1. Moisturizing and Hydration

Humectant Properties:

- **Moisture Retention:** Castor oil acts as a humectant, attracting and retaining moisture in the hair shaft. Proper hydration is essential for maintaining hair elasticity and strength, as dry hair is more susceptible to breakage.

Benefits:

- **Soft and Pliable Hair:** Well-moisturized hair is softer and more flexible, reducing the likelihood of breakage during styling and manipulation.
- **Preventing Dryness:** Hydration helps prevent hair from becoming brittle and dry, common causes of hair weakness and breakage.

2. Nutrient-Rich Composition

Essential Fatty Acids:

- **Ricinoleic Acid:** This fatty acid, which makes up about 85-90% of castor oil, nourishes the hair follicles, promoting healthier and stronger hair growth.
- **Other Fatty Acids:** Oleic acid and linoleic acid also contribute to the nutritional profile of castor oil, supporting overall hair health.

Vitamins and Minerals:

- **Vitamin E:** An antioxidant that protects hair from oxidative stress and environmental damage, enhancing hair strength and resilience.

Benefits:

- **Nourishment:** The nutrients in castor oil penetrate the hair shaft, providing deep nourishment that supports hair strength from within.
- **Resilience:** Regular use of castor oil helps fortify the hair, making it more resilient to physical and environmental stressors.

3. Sealing the Hair Cuticle

Cuticle Smoothing:

- **Protective Barrier:** Castor oil helps to smooth and seal the hair cuticle, the outermost layer of the hair shaft. A well-sealed cuticle protects the inner layers of the hair, retaining moisture and preventing damage.

Benefits:

- **Reduced Frizz:** Sealing the cuticle reduces frizz and prevents the hair from becoming rough and unmanageable.
- **Enhanced Shine:** A smooth cuticle reflects light better, giving hair a natural shine and healthier appearance.
- **Protection Against Damage:** A sealed cuticle protects hair from environmental damage, such as UV rays and pollution, which can weaken the hair structure.

4. Improving Hair Elasticity

Elasticity Enhancement:

- **Hydration and Conditioning:** The moisturizing properties of castor oil improve hair elasticity, making it more flexible and less prone to breakage.

Benefits:

- **Tensile Strength:** Improved elasticity enhances the hair's tensile strength, allowing it to withstand stretching and bending without breaking.
- **Resilience to Styling:** Elastic hair is better able to endure styling practices, such as brushing, combing, and heat styling, without sustaining damage.

5. Repairing Damage

Damage Repair:

- **Protein Retention:** Castor oil helps reduce protein loss from the hair, which is crucial for maintaining hair strength. Protein loss can lead to weakened hair that is more susceptible to breakage.

Benefits:

- **Reinforcement:** By retaining protein within the hair shaft, castor oil reinforces the hair structure, making it stronger and more durable.
- **Damage Reversal:** Regular use of castor oil can help repair damage caused by chemical treatments, heat styling, and environmental exposure.

6. Enhancing Hair Growth

Stronger Hair Growth:

- **Scalp Stimulation:** Castor oil stimulates blood circulation to the scalp, providing hair follicles with essential nutrients and oxygen that promote strong, healthy hair growth.

Benefits:

- **Thicker Hair:** Stimulating the scalp encourages the growth of thicker, more robust hair strands.
- **Root Strength:** Stronger hair starts at the roots, and castor oil helps ensure that new hair growth is healthy and resilient.

7. Anti-Inflammatory and Antimicrobial Properties

Scalp Health:

- **Reducing Inflammation:** The anti-inflammatory properties of ricinoleic acid in castor oil help soothe the scalp, reducing conditions that can weaken hair, such as dandruff and scalp irritation.
- **Preventing Infections:** Castor oil's antimicrobial properties help prevent scalp infections that can lead to hair loss and weakened hair.

Benefits:

- **Healthy Scalp Environment:** A healthy scalp is essential for strong hair growth. By maintaining scalp health, castor oil supports the overall strength and resilience of hair.
- **Reduced Hair Loss:** Preventing scalp issues reduces hair loss and promotes the growth of strong, healthy hair.

Moisturizing and Conditioning

Hydration benefits

One of the standout benefits of castor oil for hair is its exceptional moisturizing and conditioning properties. Proper hydration is crucial for maintaining healthy hair, as it prevents dryness, reduces frizz, and enhances the overall texture and appearance of the hair. Here, we explore how castor oil provides hydration benefits, its mechanisms of action, and the positive impact it has on hair health.

1. Deep Moisturization

Humectant Properties:

- **Moisture Attraction:** Castor oil is a natural humectant, meaning it attracts and retains moisture from the environment. When applied to the hair and scalp, it helps draw in moisture and lock it in, ensuring long-lasting hydration.

Benefits:

- **Prevents Dryness:** By retaining moisture, castor oil prevents the hair from becoming dry and brittle, which is essential for maintaining hair strength and elasticity.
- **Hydrated Scalp:** A well-moisturized scalp is less prone to dryness, flaking, and irritation, creating a healthy environment for hair growth.

2. Sealing the Cuticle

Cuticle Smoothing:

- **Protective Layer:** Castor oil helps to smooth and seal the hair cuticle, the outermost layer of the hair shaft. A well-sealed cuticle retains moisture better, preventing water loss and keeping the hair hydrated.

Benefits:

- **Enhanced Shine:** Sealing the cuticle adds shine to the hair by creating a smooth surface that reflects light.
- **Reduced Frizz:** A sealed cuticle reduces frizz and flyaways, making hair more manageable and easier to style.

3. Nutrient-Rich Composition

Fatty Acids:

- **Ricinoleic Acid:** The high concentration of ricinoleic acid in castor oil provides deep nourishment and hydration to the hair and scalp.
- **Oleic and Linoleic Acids:** These fatty acids contribute to the oil's moisturizing properties, ensuring that the hair remains soft and supple.

Vitamins and Antioxidants:

- **Vitamin E:** An antioxidant that helps maintain the integrity of the hair and scalp, supporting hydration and preventing damage from free radicals.

Benefits:

- **Softness and Manageability:** The nutrients in castor oil help improve the texture of the hair, making it softer, smoother, and easier to manage.

- **Healthier Hair:** Proper nourishment supports overall hair health, enhancing its appearance and resilience.

4. Conditioning Properties

Deep Conditioning Treatment:

- **Penetrative Ability:** Castor oil penetrates deeply into the hair shaft, providing intense conditioning that strengthens and revitalizes the hair from within.

Benefits:

- **Improved Elasticity:** Deep conditioning helps improve the elasticity of the hair, making it more resilient to stretching and styling.
- **Damage Repair:** Regular conditioning with castor oil can help repair damage caused by chemical treatments, heat styling, and environmental exposure.

5. Scalp Health

Hydrating the Scalp:

- **Moisture Balance:** Castor oil helps balance the moisture levels of the scalp, preventing it from becoming too dry or too oily.

Benefits:

- **Reduced Flaking:** A hydrated scalp reduces flaking and dandruff, which can impede hair growth and overall scalp health.
- **Soothed Irritation:** The moisturizing properties of castor oil soothe scalp irritation and inflammation, creating a healthier environment for hair follicles.

6. Protection Against Environmental Damage

Environmental Shielding:

- **Barrier Formation:** Castor oil forms a protective barrier on the hair shaft, shielding it from environmental factors such as pollution, UV rays, and harsh weather conditions.

Benefits:

- **Reduced Damage:** Protecting the hair from environmental damage helps maintain its health and appearance, preventing dryness and brittleness.
- **Longevity of Hair Color:** For those with color-treated hair, the protective barrier helps preserve hair color and prevent fading.

7. Enhancing Hair Texture

Smoothing Effect:

- **Frizz Control:** Castor oil's ability to smooth the hair cuticle and retain moisture reduces frizz and enhances the hair's natural texture.

Benefits:

- **Defined Curls and Waves:** For those with curly or wavy hair, castor oil helps define curls and waves, making them more pronounced and manageable.
- **Sleek Appearance:** Straight and wavy hair types benefit from a sleek, polished appearance with reduced flyaways and frizz.

Conclusion

Castor oil's moisturizing and conditioning properties make it an invaluable addition to any hair care routine. Its ability to attract and retain moisture, seal the hair cuticle, and provide deep nourishment ensures that hair remains hydrated, soft, and healthy. By improving scalp health, protecting against environmental damage, and enhancing hair texture, castor oil supports overall hair resilience and vitality. Understanding these hydration benefits highlights why castor oil is a go-to natural remedy for achieving and maintaining beautiful, healthy hair.

Comparison with other conditioners

Castor oil is a highly effective natural conditioner, but how does it compare to other popular conditioning agents? Each type of conditioner, whether natural or synthetic, has unique properties and benefits. Here, we compare castor oil with other common conditioners to highlight their differences and advantages in hair care.

1. Castor Oil

Properties:

- **Natural Humectant:** Attracts and retains moisture.
- **High in Ricinoleic Acid:** Provides anti-inflammatory and antimicrobial benefits.
- **Thick Consistency:** Penetrates deeply into the hair shaft for intense hydration.

Benefits:

- **Deep Moisturization:** Provides long-lasting hydration, preventing dryness and brittleness.
- **Scalp Health:** Promotes a healthy scalp environment, reducing dandruff and irritation.
- **Hair Strength:** Strengthens hair from within, reducing breakage and enhancing overall health.

Best For:

- **Dry and Brittle Hair:** Ideal for deeply hydrating and softening hair.
- **Damaged Hair:** Excellent for repairing and conditioning damaged hair.
- **All Hair Types:** Versatile enough for all hair types, including thick, coarse hair.

2. Coconut Oil

Properties:

- **Penetrating Ability:** Penetrates the hair shaft more effectively than many other oils.
- **Lauric Acid:** Contains high levels of lauric acid, which has antimicrobial properties.
- **Lightweight:** Lighter consistency compared to castor oil.

Benefits:

- **Protein Loss Prevention:** Helps reduce protein loss from hair during washing and conditioning.
- **Scalp Health:** Antimicrobial properties help maintain a healthy scalp.
- **Smoothness and Shine:** Adds shine and smoothness to hair, reducing frizz.

Best For:

- **Fine to Medium Hair:** Suitable for fine to medium hair types that need light, non-greasy hydration.
- **Damaged Hair:** Effective for repairing damaged hair due to its protein-retaining properties.
- **Daily Use:** Can be used regularly without weighing down the hair.

3. Argan Oil

Properties:

- **Rich in Vitamin E:** High levels of vitamin E and fatty acids.
- **Lightweight:** Lightweight and easily absorbed by the hair.
- **Antioxidant:** Contains antioxidants that protect hair from damage.

Benefits:

- **Frizz Control:** Reduces frizz and adds shine.
- **Moisturization:** Provides lightweight hydration without making hair greasy.
- **Protection:** Protects hair from environmental damage and UV rays.

Best For:

- **Frizzy Hair:** Ideal for controlling frizz and adding shine.
- **Color-Treated Hair:** Helps preserve color and prevent fading.
- **Daily Conditioning:** Suitable for daily use due to its lightweight nature.

4. Shea Butter

Properties:

- **Intensive Moisturizer:** Rich and creamy texture.
- **Vitamins and Fatty Acids:** High in vitamins A and E, and essential fatty acids.
- **Emollient:** Excellent emollient properties.

Benefits:

- **Deep Conditioning:** Provides intense hydration and nourishment.
- **Protection:** Forms a protective barrier that locks in moisture.
- **Scalp Health:** Soothes dry and irritated scalp conditions.

Best For:

- **Thick, Coarse Hair:** Ideal for thick, coarse, and curly hair types.
- **Dry, Damaged Hair:** Excellent for deeply conditioning and repairing dry, damaged hair.
- **Protective Styling:** Suitable for use in protective hairstyles to prevent breakage.

5. Jojoba Oil

Properties:

- **Similar to Sebum:** Closely resembles the natural sebum produced by the scalp.
- **Lightweight:** Non-greasy and easily absorbed.
- **Balancing:** Helps balance oil production on the scalp.

Benefits:

- **Scalp Health:** Balances oil production, making it ideal for both dry and oily scalps.
- **Light Moisturization:** Provides light, non-greasy hydration.
- **Nourishing:** Nourishes the scalp and hair without weighing it down.

Best For:

- **Oily Hair:** Ideal for those with oily hair and scalp, as it helps regulate sebum production.
- **Sensitive Scalp:** Suitable for sensitive scalps due to its gentle, non-irritating properties.
- **Fine Hair:** Great for fine hair that needs lightweight conditioning.

6. Commercial Synthetic Conditioners

Properties:

- **Varied Ingredients:** Contain a mix of silicones, proteins, and moisturizing agents.
- **Immediate Results:** Often provide immediate smoothness and detangling.

- **Silicones:** Commonly contain silicones for a smooth, shiny finish.

Benefits:

- **Detangling:** Excellent for detangling hair and reducing friction.
- **Instant Smoothness:** Provide immediate results in terms of smoothness and manageability.
- **Variety:** Available for various hair types and specific hair concerns.

Best For:

- **Convenience:** Ideal for those looking for quick and easy hair care solutions.
- **Specific Hair Issues:** Formulated to address specific hair issues such as frizz, volume, or color protection.
- **Temporary Results:** Suitable for immediate, short-term improvements in hair appearance.

Treating Scalp Conditions

Scalp health improvement

Healthy hair starts with a healthy scalp. Castor oil is highly effective in treating various scalp conditions due to its unique composition and properties. By addressing issues such as dandruff, scalp inflammation, and infections, castor oil helps create an optimal environment for hair growth and overall hair health. Here, we explore how castor oil improves scalp health and treats common scalp conditions.

1. Anti-Inflammatory Properties

Ricinoleic Acid:

- **Inflammation Reduction:** Ricinoleic acid, the primary fatty acid in castor oil, has potent anti-inflammatory properties. It helps reduce inflammation on the scalp, which can be caused by conditions like seborrheic dermatitis, psoriasis, and eczema.

Benefits:

- **Soothe Irritation:** Reduces redness, itching, and irritation, providing relief from discomfort.
- **Promote Healing:** Encourages the healing of inflamed and irritated scalp areas, restoring a healthy scalp environment.

2. Antimicrobial Action

Antibacterial and Antifungal Properties:

- **Infection Prevention:** Castor oil's antimicrobial properties help prevent and treat scalp infections caused by bacteria and fungi. This includes conditions like dandruff, folliculitis, and ringworm.

Benefits:

- **Combat Dandruff:** Helps control dandruff by addressing the fungal infection (Malassezia) often responsible for flaking and itching.
- **Healthy Scalp Environment:** Maintains a clean and infection-free scalp, which is crucial for healthy hair growth.

3. Moisturizing and Hydration

Humectant Properties:

- **Moisture Retention:** Castor oil acts as a humectant, attracting and retaining moisture in the scalp. Proper hydration is essential for preventing dryness and flakiness.

Benefits:

- **Prevent Dry Scalp:** Keeps the scalp moisturized, reducing dryness and the risk of flaking.
- **Nourish and Hydrate:** Provides deep hydration, which is essential for maintaining a healthy scalp and supporting hair growth.

4. Balancing Scalp Oil Production

Sebum Regulation:

- **Oil Balance:** Castor oil helps regulate the production of sebum, the natural oil produced by the scalp. It ensures that the scalp is neither too oily nor too dry.

Benefits:

- **Prevent Excess Oil:** Reduces excess oil production, which can clog hair follicles and lead to scalp issues.
- **Moisture Balance:** Maintains a balanced level of moisture, preventing both dryness and greasiness.

5. Exfoliation and Detoxification

Scalp Cleansing:

- **Detoxifying:** Castor oil can help cleanse and detoxify the scalp by removing impurities, dead skin cells, and excess oil.

Benefits:

- **Unclog Pores:** Keeps hair follicles unclogged, promoting healthy hair growth.
- **Refresh Scalp:** Leaves the scalp feeling refreshed and rejuvenated, reducing the buildup of products and pollutants.

6. Stimulating Blood Circulation

Scalp Stimulation:

- **Improved Circulation:** Massaging castor oil into the scalp stimulates blood circulation, ensuring that hair follicles receive adequate nutrients and oxygen.

Benefits:

- **Nutrient Delivery:** Enhanced blood flow delivers essential nutrients to the hair follicles, supporting their health and function.
- **Healthy Hair Growth:** Improved circulation promotes healthy hair growth by providing a better environment for hair follicles.

7. Soothing and Calming Effect

Soothing Sensation:

- **Comfort and Relief:** The thick, rich consistency of castor oil provides a soothing and calming effect on the scalp, offering relief from irritation and discomfort.

Benefits:

- **Relaxation:** Provides a relaxing experience when massaged into the scalp, reducing stress and tension.
- **Scalp Comfort:** Offers immediate comfort for irritated or inflamed scalp conditions.

8. Strengthening Hair Roots

Root Strengthening:

- **Fortifying Hair Roots:** Castor oil strengthens hair roots, reducing hair fall and breakage associated with scalp conditions.

Benefits:

- **Reduced Hair Loss:** Strengthening the roots helps reduce hair fall caused by weak or damaged follicles.
- **Robust Hair Growth:** Ensures that new hair growth is strong and healthy.

Examples of conditions treated

Castor oil is a versatile natural remedy that can effectively treat a variety of scalp conditions. Its unique properties, including anti-inflammatory, antimicrobial, and moisturizing effects, make it particularly beneficial for improving scalp health and promoting hair growth. Here, we explore specific scalp conditions that can be treated with castor oil and explain how it helps manage and alleviate these issues.

1. Dandruff

Condition Overview:

- **Symptoms:** Dandruff is characterized by white flakes of dead skin on the scalp and in the hair, often accompanied by itching and irritation.
- **Causes:** Commonly caused by an overgrowth of the yeast-like fungus Malassezia, excessive oil production, or sensitivity to hair care products.

How Castor Oil Helps:

- **Antifungal Properties:** The antifungal properties of castor oil help control the growth of Malassezia, reducing dandruff and its associated symptoms.
- **Moisturization:** Castor oil hydrates the scalp, preventing dryness and flakiness that contribute to dandruff.
- **Soothing Effect:** Its anti-inflammatory properties soothe scalp irritation and itching.

2. Seborrheic Dermatitis

Condition Overview:

- **Symptoms:** Seborrheic dermatitis causes red, greasy, and scaly patches on the scalp, often accompanied by dandruff and itching.
- **Causes:** This condition is thought to be related to an overactive sebaceous gland and the presence of Malassezia yeast.

How Castor Oil Helps:

- **Anti-Inflammatory:** Ricinoleic acid in castor oil reduces inflammation and redness associated with seborrheic dermatitis.
- **Antimicrobial:** The antimicrobial properties help control fungal growth, reducing symptoms.
- **Oil Regulation:** Castor oil helps balance the production of sebum, preventing excessive oiliness that can exacerbate the condition.

3. Psoriasis

Condition Overview:

- **Symptoms:** Psoriasis on the scalp manifests as red, scaly patches that can be itchy and sometimes painful.
- **Causes:** An autoimmune disorder that accelerates the growth cycle of skin cells, leading to buildup and inflammation.

How Castor Oil Helps:

- **Moisturization:** Castor oil deeply moisturizes the scalp, helping to soften and remove scales.
- **Anti-Inflammatory:** Reduces inflammation and soothes irritated skin.
- **Healing Promotion:** Encourages healing of the affected skin areas.

4. Folliculitis

Condition Overview:

- **Symptoms:** Folliculitis is the inflammation of hair follicles, resulting in red, bumpy, and often itchy or painful lesions on the scalp.
- **Causes:** Usually caused by bacterial or fungal infections, friction, or irritation from hair care products.

How Castor Oil Helps:

- **Antibacterial and Antifungal:** The antimicrobial properties of castor oil help treat and prevent infections that cause folliculitis.
- **Soothing Effect:** Reduces itching and discomfort associated with folliculitis.
- **Healing:** Promotes healing of the inflamed follicles, reducing the appearance of lesions.

5. Scalp Eczema (Atopic Dermatitis)

Condition Overview:

- **Symptoms:** Scalp eczema causes dry, itchy, and inflamed skin on the scalp, often with red patches.
- **Causes:** A chronic condition often triggered by allergens, irritants, or stress.

How Castor Oil Helps:

- **Moisturization:** Keeps the scalp hydrated, preventing dryness and flaking.
- **Anti-Inflammatory:** Reduces inflammation and soothes the itchy, irritated scalp.
- **Barrier Protection:** Forms a protective barrier on the scalp, shielding it from irritants.

6. Scalp Dryness

Condition Overview:

- **Symptoms:** Scalp dryness is characterized by tight, itchy skin and flaking, often mistaken for dandruff.
- **Causes:** Can result from harsh weather, overuse of styling products, or washing hair with hot water.

How Castor Oil Helps:

- **Deep Moisturization:** Hydrates the scalp, restoring its natural moisture balance.
- **Soothing:** Relieves itching and discomfort associated with dryness.
- **Protective Layer:** Forms a protective barrier that locks in moisture and prevents further dryness.

7. Alopecia Areata

Condition Overview:

- **Symptoms:** An autoimmune condition that causes patchy hair loss on the scalp and other parts of the body.
- **Causes:** The immune system mistakenly attacks hair follicles, leading to hair loss.

How Castor Oil Helps:

- **Scalp Stimulation:** Massaging castor oil into the scalp improves blood circulation, promoting hair growth.
- **Anti-Inflammatory:** Reduces inflammation around the hair follicles.
- **Nourishment:** Provides essential nutrients that support hair follicle health and regeneration.

8. Ringworm (Tinea Capitis)

Condition Overview:

- **Symptoms:** Ringworm of the scalp is a fungal infection that causes red, scaly, and itchy patches, sometimes with hair loss in the affected areas.
- **Causes:** Caused by a dermatophyte fungus.

How Castor Oil Helps:

- **Antifungal Properties:** Castor oil's antifungal properties help treat and prevent fungal infections like ringworm.
- **Soothing:** Relieves itching and discomfort.
- **Healing:** Promotes the healing of affected areas and helps restore hair growth in the infected patches.

How to Choose the Right Castor Oil

Cold-Pressed vs. Refined

Differences and benefits

Selecting the right type of castor oil is crucial for maximizing its benefits for hair care. The two primary types are cold-pressed and refined castor oil. Each type has distinct characteristics, extraction processes, and benefits. Understanding these differences can help you make an informed decision based on your specific needs. Here, we explore the differences and benefits of cold-pressed and refined castor oil.

1. Cold-Pressed Castor Oil

Extraction Process:

- **Mechanical Pressing:** Cold-pressed castor oil is extracted by mechanically pressing castor beans without applying heat. This method preserves the oil's natural nutrients and properties.

Characteristics:

- **Natural and Pure:** Retains most of the original nutrients, including vitamins, fatty acids, and antioxidants.
- **Light Color:** Typically has a pale yellow color.
- **Distinctive Odor:** May have a mild, natural odor due to the absence of heat processing.

Benefits:

- **Nutrient-Rich:** High in ricinoleic acid, vitamin E, and essential fatty acids, making it highly beneficial for hair and scalp health.
- **Hydration:** Provides excellent hydration, keeping hair moisturized and preventing dryness and brittleness.
- **Scalp Health:** The natural nutrients help maintain a healthy scalp, reducing dandruff and irritation.
- **Hair Strength:** Strengthens hair from within, reducing breakage and enhancing overall hair health.
- **Chemical-Free:** Free from chemicals and additives, making it ideal for sensitive scalps and those looking for a natural product.

Best For:

- **Sensitive Scalps:** Ideal for individuals with sensitive scalps or those prone to allergies.
- **Natural Hair Care:** Suitable for those who prefer organic and natural products in their hair care routine.

- **General Hair Health:** Provides the necessary nutrients for maintaining healthy hair and scalp.

2. Refined Castor Oil

Extraction Process:

- **Refinement:** Refined castor oil undergoes processing to remove impurities, color, and odor. This involves filtration and bleaching to produce a more aesthetically pleasing product.

Characteristics:

- **Processed:** Undergoes additional processing to remove impurities and enhance its appearance.
- **Light Color:** Has a lighter color compared to unrefined castor oil.
- **Mild Odor:** Possesses a mild odor due to the refinement process.

Benefits:

- **Cosmetic Use:** Often used in cosmetic formulations due to its light color and mild odor, making it suitable for a wide range of products.
- **Versatile:** Suitable for various hair care applications, including conditioning and styling.
- **Smooth Application:** The refinement process can make the oil smoother and easier to apply.

Best For:

- **Cosmetic Formulations:** Ideal for inclusion in DIY hair care products and cosmetic formulations.
- **Sensitive Users:** Suitable for those who are sensitive to strong smells or prefer a lighter oil.
- **General Hair Care:** Can be used for regular hair conditioning and maintenance.

3. Comparison of Cold-Pressed vs. Refined Castor Oil

Nutrient Content:

- **Cold-Pressed:** Retains most of the original nutrients, making it more beneficial for hair and scalp health.
- **Refined:** Some nutrients may be lost during the refinement process, but it still retains beneficial properties.

Color and Odor:

- **Cold-Pressed:** Has a pale yellow color and a distinctive, natural odor.
- **Refined:** Typically lighter in color with a milder odor, making it more aesthetically pleasing for cosmetic use.

Purity:

- **Cold-Pressed:** Generally considered more natural and pure, free from chemicals and additives.
- **Refined:** Undergoes processing to remove impurities, which can make it less pure but more stable and suitable for certain applications.

Application:

- **Cold-Pressed:** Ideal for direct application to the hair and scalp, providing maximum benefits from its rich nutrient content.
- **Refined:** Suitable for use in various hair care products and formulations, offering a smoother application experience.

4. Making the Right Choice

Consider Your Needs:

- **Hair and Scalp Health:** If your primary goal is to improve hair and scalp health, cold-pressed castor oil is the best choice due to its high nutrient content and natural properties.
- **Cosmetic and DIY Products:** If you plan to use castor oil in DIY hair care products or prefer a lighter, milder oil, refined castor oil is more suitable.

Check for Certifications:

- **Organic Certification:** Look for organic certifications if you prefer a product free from synthetic chemicals and pesticides.
- **Cold-Pressed Certification:** Ensure the product is certified as cold-pressed to guarantee its nutrient retention and purity.

Read Labels:

- **Ingredient List:** Check the ingredient list to ensure the product does not contain unnecessary additives or chemicals.
- **Source Information:** Verify the source of the castor oil to ensure it is of high quality and sustainably produced.

Recommendations for hair care

Choosing the right castor oil is crucial for maximizing its benefits for hair care. Here are specific recommendations to guide you in selecting the best type of castor oil for various hair care needs.

1. For Dry and Brittle Hair

Cold-Pressed Castor Oil:

- **Reason:** Cold-pressed castor oil retains the most nutrients, including ricinoleic acid, vitamin E, and essential fatty acids, which provide deep moisturization and nourishment.
- **Application:** Apply directly to the hair and scalp as a deep conditioning treatment. Use it as an overnight mask or a weekly treatment to restore moisture and reduce brittleness.

Recommendation:

- **Frequency:** Use 2-3 times a week for best results.
- **Method:** Massage a small amount of oil into the scalp and distribute through the hair. Cover with a shower cap and leave on overnight, then wash out thoroughly in the morning.

2. For Oily Scalp and Hair

Jojoba Oil with Castor Oil:

- **Reason:** Jojoba oil closely resembles the scalp's natural sebum and helps regulate oil production. When mixed with castor oil, it provides balanced moisturization without making the hair greasy.
- **Application:** Mix equal parts of jojoba oil and castor oil. Apply to the scalp and hair, focusing on the roots.

Recommendation:

- **Frequency:** Use once a week to avoid overloading the scalp with oil.
- **Method:** Massage the mixture into the scalp, leave on for 30 minutes to an hour, then wash out with a mild shampoo.

3. For Scalp Conditions (Dandruff, Seborrheic Dermatitis, Psoriasis)

Cold-Pressed or Jamaican Black Castor Oil:

- **Reason:** Both types of castor oil have antifungal, antibacterial, and anti-inflammatory properties that help treat scalp conditions.
- **Application:** Use castor oil as a scalp treatment to reduce inflammation, control fungal growth, and soothe irritation.

Recommendation:

- **Frequency:** Apply 2-3 times a week for severe conditions, then reduce to once a week for maintenance.
- **Method:** Massage the oil into the scalp, focusing on affected areas. Leave on for at least an hour before washing out. For best results, use a gentle, anti-dandruff shampoo.

4. For Hair Growth and Thickness

Cold-Pressed or Jamaican Black Castor Oil:

- **Reason:** Both types are highly effective in stimulating hair growth and increasing hair thickness due to their nutrient-rich composition and ability to improve blood circulation to the scalp.
- **Application:** Use as a scalp massage oil to stimulate hair follicles and promote growth.

Recommendation:

- **Frequency:** Use 2-3 times a week.
- **Method:** Warm a small amount of oil and massage it into the scalp in circular motions for 5-10 minutes. Leave on for at least an hour or overnight for better results, then wash out.

5. For Damaged Hair

Cold-Pressed Castor Oil with Coconut Oil:

- **Reason:** Combining castor oil with coconut oil enhances its ability to repair damaged hair by providing additional nutrients and deep moisturization.
- **Application:** Mix equal parts of cold-pressed castor oil and coconut oil. Use as a deep conditioning treatment to repair and strengthen damaged hair.

Recommendation:

- **Frequency:** Use once a week as a deep conditioning treatment.
- **Method:** Apply the mixture to the hair, focusing on the ends and damaged areas. Cover with a shower cap and leave on for at least an hour or overnight, then wash out thoroughly.

6. For Fine or Thin Hair

Lightweight Oil Blend:

- **Reason:** Fine or thin hair can benefit from a lighter oil blend that won't weigh the hair down. Mixing castor oil with lighter oils like argan or grapeseed oil provides the benefits of castor oil without the heaviness.
- **Application:** Mix castor oil with argan or grapeseed oil in a ratio of 1:2. Apply sparingly to avoid weighing down the hair.

Recommendation:

- **Frequency:** Use once a week.
- **Method:** Apply a small amount of the blend to the scalp and hair, focusing on the roots. Leave on for 30 minutes to an hour, then wash out with a gentle shampoo.

7. For Regular Hair Maintenance

Cold-Pressed Castor Oil:

- **Reason:** Cold-pressed castor oil provides the necessary nutrients for maintaining overall hair health, including moisture, strength, and scalp health.
- **Application:** Use as a regular treatment to keep hair healthy and strong.

Recommendation:

- **Frequency:** Use once a week for regular maintenance.
- **Method:** Apply a small amount to the scalp and hair, leave on for 30 minutes to an hour, then wash out with a mild shampoo.

Organic vs. Non-Organic

Importance of organic options

When choosing castor oil for hair care, one of the important considerations is whether to opt for organic or non-organic varieties. Organic castor oil is produced without the use of synthetic pesticides, fertilizers, or genetically modified organisms (GMOs), ensuring a purer and more natural product. Here, we explore the differences between organic and non-organic castor oil, and why choosing organic options can be beneficial for your hair and overall health.

1. Organic Castor Oil

Production Process:

- **Natural Farming Practices:** Organic castor oil is derived from castor beans grown without synthetic pesticides, fertilizers, or GMOs. Organic farming practices focus on sustainability, soil health, and environmental protection.
- **Certification:** To be labeled as organic, castor oil must meet specific certification standards set by regulatory bodies, such as USDA Organic or EU Organic.

Characteristics:

- **Chemical-Free:** Free from synthetic chemicals and additives.
- **Nutrient-Rich:** Retains natural nutrients due to the absence of chemical processing.
- **Sustainable:** Produced through environmentally friendly farming practices.

Benefits:

- **Healthier Scalp and Hair:** Organic castor oil is free from harmful chemicals that can irritate the scalp and damage hair. It provides a purer, more natural option for hair care.

- **Environmental Impact:** Organic farming practices reduce environmental pollution and promote biodiversity. By choosing organic castor oil, you support sustainable agriculture and environmental conservation.
- **Better Nutrient Profile:** Organic castor oil tends to retain more of its natural nutrients, including vitamins, fatty acids, and antioxidants, which are beneficial for hair health.

Best For:

- **Sensitive Scalps:** Ideal for individuals with sensitive scalps or those prone to allergic reactions.
- **Natural Hair Care:** Suitable for those who prefer organic and natural products in their hair care routine.
- **Sustainable Choices:** Great for consumers who are environmentally conscious and prefer sustainable products.

2. Non-Organic Castor Oil

Production Process:

- **Conventional Farming:** Non-organic castor oil is derived from castor beans grown using conventional farming methods, which may include synthetic pesticides, fertilizers, and GMOs.
- **Processing:** The oil may undergo additional processing to remove impurities, which can sometimes involve the use of chemicals.

Characteristics:

- **May Contain Residues:** Can contain residues of synthetic chemicals used during farming and processing.
- **Varied Nutrient Content:** Nutrient content may be lower due to chemical exposure and processing methods.
- **Widely Available:** More readily available and often less expensive than organic options.

Benefits:

- **Cost-Effective:** Generally less expensive than organic castor oil, making it a budget-friendly option.
- **Availability:** Easier to find in stores and online due to its widespread production.

Best For:

- **Budget-Conscious Consumers:** Suitable for those who are looking for a cost-effective option for hair care.
- **General Use:** Can be used for general hair care needs if budget is a primary concern.

3. Importance of Choosing Organic Castor Oil

Health and Safety:

- **Chemical-Free:** Organic castor oil is free from potentially harmful synthetic chemicals, reducing the risk of scalp irritation, allergic reactions, and long-term health effects.
- **Purer Product:** Ensures a purer, more natural product that is safer for both the scalp and hair.

Environmental Sustainability:

- **Eco-Friendly Practices:** Organic farming practices are designed to be environmentally friendly, promoting soil health, reducing pollution, and supporting biodiversity.
- **Sustainable Agriculture:** By choosing organic products, consumers support sustainable agricultural practices that are better for the planet.

Nutrient Density:

- **Higher Nutrient Content:** Organic castor oil often retains more of its natural nutrients, providing better nourishment for the hair and scalp.
- **Enhanced Benefits:** The higher nutrient density translates to enhanced benefits for hair health, including better hydration, reduced breakage, and improved overall hair strength.

Ethical Considerations:

- **Fair Trade and Ethical Practices:** Many organic products are also produced under fair trade conditions, ensuring that farmers and workers are paid fairly and work in safe conditions.
- **Supporting Small Farms:** Choosing organic often supports small, local farms that practice sustainable agriculture.

Reading Labels and Certifications

How to interpret product labels

Choosing the right castor oil for hair care involves understanding the information provided on product labels and certifications. Properly interpreting these labels can help you make informed decisions, ensuring you select high-quality products that meet your needs. Here, we explore how to read and understand product labels and certifications for castor oil.

1. Ingredient List

Key Points:

- **Single Ingredient:** Ideally, the ingredient list for castor oil should be short, listing only "Ricinus Communis (Castor) Seed Oil." This indicates that the product is pure castor oil without additives.
- **Additives and Fillers:** If the ingredient list includes other ingredients, such as fragrances, preservatives, or fillers, it means the product is not 100% pure castor oil. While some additives can be beneficial, others might not be necessary and could cause irritation for sensitive users.

How to Read:

- **First Ingredient:** The first ingredient listed is usually the primary component of the product. Ensure that "Ricinus Communis (Castor) Seed Oil" is the first and ideally the only ingredient.
- **Additives:** Look for any additional ingredients. Understand their purpose and decide if they are necessary for your hair care routine. Avoid products with unnecessary or potentially harmful additives.

2. Certifications

Organic Certifications:

- **USDA Organic:** Indicates the product is certified organic by the United States Department of Agriculture. This certification ensures that the castor beans were grown without synthetic pesticides, fertilizers, or GMOs.
- **EU Organic:** Similar to USDA Organic, this certification is provided by the European Union and ensures the product meets EU organic farming standards.
- **Other Certifications:** Look for other reputable organic certifications, such as EcoCert, which also guarantee that the product meets organic farming standards.

Fair Trade Certification:

- **Fair Trade Certified:** Indicates that the product was produced under fair trade conditions, ensuring that farmers and workers were paid fairly and worked in safe conditions. This certification supports ethical sourcing and sustainable practices.

Non-GMO Certification:

- **Non-GMO Project Verified:** Ensures that the product does not contain genetically modified organisms. This is important for consumers who prefer natural and non-GMO products.

How to Read:

- **Certification Seals:** Look for certification seals on the product packaging. These seals provide assurance that the product meets specific standards.

- **Certification Details:** Understand what each certification means and how it aligns with your values and needs. Choose products with certifications that guarantee quality, safety, and ethical production.

3. Product Descriptions

Cold-Pressed vs. Refined:

- **Cold-Pressed:** Look for labels that indicate the oil is cold-pressed. This extraction method preserves the natural nutrients and benefits of the castor oil.
- **Refined:** If the label indicates that the oil is refined, it means the oil has undergone additional processing to remove impurities, which can affect its nutrient content and purity.

Hexane-Free:

- **Hexane-Free:** Ensure the label specifies that the product is hexane-free. Hexane is a solvent sometimes used in the extraction process, but it can leave residues in the oil. Hexane-free products are purer and safer for hair care.

100% Pure:

- **Pure Castor Oil:** Look for labels that state the product is 100% pure castor oil. This ensures that you are getting an undiluted product with all its natural benefits intact.

How to Read:

- **Extraction Method:** Verify the extraction method indicated on the label (cold-pressed or refined). Cold-pressed is generally preferred for hair care due to its higher nutrient retention.
- **Purity Claims:** Ensure the label claims the product is 100% pure and hexane-free for the highest quality and safety.

4. Shelf Life and Storage

Expiration Date:

- **Check Expiry:** Always check the expiration date on the label to ensure the product is fresh. Using expired oil can reduce its effectiveness and potentially cause irritation.

Storage Instructions:

- **Proper Storage:** Look for storage instructions to maintain the oil's quality. Typically, castor oil should be stored in a cool, dark place to prevent it from going rancid.

How to Read:

- **Expiry Date:** Confirm the product is within its shelf life before purchase.
- **Storage Tips:** Follow any storage instructions provided to maintain the oil's efficacy.

5. Brand Transparency

Reputable Brands:

- **Research Brands:** Choose products from reputable brands known for their quality and transparency. Research the brand's sourcing practices, production methods, and overall reputation.
- **Transparency:** Brands that provide detailed information about their sourcing and production processes are often more trustworthy.

Customer Reviews:

- **Read Reviews:** Check customer reviews to gauge the product's effectiveness and any potential issues. Reviews can provide insights into the product's real-world performance.

How to Read:

- **Brand Information:** Look for brands that are transparent about their processes and ingredients.
- **Customer Feedback:** Consider feedback from other users to make an informed decision.

Trusted certifications and what they mean

Choosing castor oil with trusted certifications ensures you are getting a high-quality, safe, and ethically produced product. These certifications provide assurance about the oil's purity, organic status, non-GMO status, and ethical production practices. Here, we explore some of the most trusted certifications for castor oil and what they signify.

1. USDA Organic

Certification Overview:

- **USDA Organic:** The United States Department of Agriculture (USDA) Organic certification indicates that the product meets stringent organic farming standards set by the USDA. This includes the prohibition of synthetic pesticides, fertilizers, and GMOs.

What It Means:

- **Chemical-Free:** The castor oil is free from synthetic chemicals and additives, making it safer for use on hair and skin.
- **Sustainable Farming:** The castor beans are grown using sustainable agricultural practices that promote soil health and biodiversity.
- **Non-GMO:** The product does not contain genetically modified organisms.

Benefits:

- **Healthier Product:** Ensures a pure and natural product that is better for your hair and scalp.
- **Environmental Impact:** Supports environmentally friendly farming practices.
- **Consumer Confidence:** Provides assurance of the product's quality and safety.

2. EU Organic

Certification Overview:

- **EU Organic:** The European Union Organic certification indicates that the product meets the EU's organic farming standards, which are similar to those of the USDA.

What It Means:

- **High Standards:** The product complies with rigorous organic standards, ensuring it is free from synthetic pesticides, fertilizers, and GMOs.
- **Traceability:** Ensures full traceability of the product from farm to shelf.

Benefits:

- **Purity:** Guarantees a chemical-free product.
- **Sustainability:** Supports sustainable farming practices in Europe.
- **Trust:** Enhances consumer trust in the product's organic integrity.

3. EcoCert

Certification Overview:

- **EcoCert:** An international organic certification body that certifies products based on strict environmental and social criteria.

What It Means:

- **Natural Ingredients:** Ensures that a significant percentage of the ingredients are natural and organic.
- **Environmental Responsibility:** Emphasizes environmentally friendly production processes and packaging.
- **Ethical Sourcing:** Ensures fair trade practices and respect for biodiversity.

Benefits:

- **Natural Assurance:** Confirms the product is made from natural and organic ingredients.
- **Eco-Friendly:** Promotes sustainable and eco-friendly production methods.
- **Ethical Practices:** Supports ethical sourcing and fair trade.

4. Non-GMO Project Verified

Certification Overview:

- **Non-GMO Project Verified:** Indicates that the product has been tested and verified to be free from genetically modified organisms.

What It Means:

- **Non-GMO:** The product does not contain genetically modified ingredients, ensuring it is natural and unaltered.
- **Testing and Verification:** Involves rigorous testing and verification processes to confirm non-GMO status.

Benefits:

- **Natural Integrity:** Ensures the product is natural and free from genetic modification.
- **Consumer Trust:** Provides assurance about the product's purity and natural origin.

5. Fair Trade Certified

Certification Overview:

- **Fair Trade Certified:** Ensures that the product was produced under fair trade conditions, supporting fair wages, safe working conditions, and community development.

What It Means:

- **Fair Wages:** Farmers and workers are paid fair wages, helping to improve their quality of life.
- **Safe Conditions:** Ensures safe and healthy working conditions for all workers involved in the production process.
- **Community Support:** Promotes community development and empowerment through fair trade practices.

Benefits:

- **Ethical Sourcing:** Supports ethical and fair trade practices.
- **Social Responsibility:** Contributes to the well-being of farming communities.
- **Consumer Ethics:** Allows consumers to make ethical purchasing decisions.

6. ISO Certification

Certification Overview:

- **ISO Certification:** Indicates that the product meets international standards set by the International Organization for Standardization (ISO) for quality, safety, and efficiency.

What It Means:

- **Quality Assurance:** Ensures the product meets high standards of quality and safety.
- **Consistency:** Promotes consistency in production processes, ensuring reliable product quality.

Benefits:

- **High Standards:** Guarantees the product is manufactured to rigorous international standards.
- **Consumer Confidence:** Enhances trust in the product's quality and safety.

7. Kosher and Halal Certifications

Certification Overview:

- **Kosher Certification:** Indicates that the product meets Jewish dietary laws and is suitable for consumption and use by individuals following kosher guidelines.
- **Halal Certification:** Indicates that the product meets Islamic dietary laws and is suitable for consumption and use by individuals following halal guidelines.

What They Mean:

- **Religious Compliance:** Ensures the product is compliant with specific religious dietary laws and practices.
- **Quality and Purity:** Confirms that the product meets high standards of quality and purity.

Benefits:

- **Inclusive:** Makes the product accessible to individuals following kosher or halal dietary laws.
- **Quality Assurance:** Provides additional assurance of the product's quality and integrity.

Part III

Practical Applications of Castor Oil

Preparation and Application Techniques

How to Prepare Castor Oil for Use

Methods of preparation

Properly preparing castor oil before application can enhance its effectiveness and ensure optimal results. Here are various methods to prepare castor oil for use in your hair care routine:

1. Direct Application

Method Overview:

- **Pure Castor Oil:** Direct application of pure castor oil is a straightforward method that involves using the oil in its natural form without any additives.

Steps:

1. **Warm the Oil:** Pour a small amount of castor oil into a bowl and warm it slightly. You can do this by placing the bowl in a larger bowl of hot water. Warm oil penetrates the hair and scalp more effectively.
2. **Apply to Scalp and Hair:** Using your fingertips, apply the warm castor oil directly to your scalp. Massage gently in circular motions to ensure even distribution. After covering the scalp, apply the oil to the length of your hair, focusing on the ends.
3. **Leave On:** Cover your hair with a shower cap and leave the oil on for at least 30 minutes. For deeper conditioning, leave it on overnight.
4. **Rinse and Shampoo:** Rinse thoroughly with lukewarm water and shampoo as usual to remove the oil.

2. Dilution with Carrier Oils

Method Overview:

- **Carrier Oil Blend:** Diluting castor oil with lighter carrier oils can make it easier to apply and less sticky, especially for those with fine or oily hair.

Steps:

1. **Choose Carrier Oils:** Select a carrier oil such as coconut oil, jojoba oil, or argan oil. These oils complement castor oil and provide additional benefits.
2. **Mix the Oils:** In a bowl, mix equal parts of castor oil and the chosen carrier oil. Adjust the ratio as needed based on your hair type and preference.
3. **Warm the Blend:** Warm the oil blend slightly by placing the bowl in a larger bowl of hot water.
4. **Apply to Scalp and Hair:** Using your fingertips, apply the warm oil blend to your scalp and massage gently. Apply the remaining oil to the length of your hair.

5. **Leave On:** Cover your hair with a shower cap and leave the oil on for at least 30 minutes or overnight for deeper conditioning.
6. **Rinse and Shampoo:** Rinse thoroughly and shampoo to remove the oil blend.

3. Infusion with Essential Oils

Method Overview:

- **Essential Oil Enhancement:** Adding a few drops of essential oils to castor oil can enhance its benefits and add a pleasant scent.

Steps:

1. **Choose Essential Oils:** Select essential oils such as rosemary, lavender, or peppermint. These oils can stimulate hair growth, soothe the scalp, and add fragrance.
2. **Mix the Oils:** In a bowl, mix 2-3 tablespoons of castor oil with 5-10 drops of your chosen essential oil.
3. **Warm the Blend:** Warm the oil blend slightly by placing the bowl in a larger bowl of hot water.
4. **Apply to Scalp and Hair:** Using your fingertips, apply the warm oil blend to your scalp and massage gently. Apply the remaining oil to the length of your hair.
5. **Leave On:** Cover your hair with a shower cap and leave the oil on for at least 30 minutes or overnight for deeper conditioning.
6. **Rinse and Shampoo:** Rinse thoroughly and shampoo to remove the oil blend.

4. DIY Hair Mask

Method Overview:

- **Nutrient-Rich Hair Mask:** Combine castor oil with other nourishing ingredients to create a DIY hair mask that provides deep conditioning and revitalization.

Steps:

1. **Gather Ingredients:** Prepare ingredients such as castor oil, honey, yogurt, and egg. These ingredients provide additional moisture, protein, and nutrients.
2. **Mix the Ingredients:** In a bowl, mix 2 tablespoons of castor oil with 1 tablespoon of honey, 2 tablespoons of yogurt, and 1 egg. Whisk until well combined.
3. **Apply the Mask:** Using your fingertips or a brush, apply the hair mask to your scalp and hair. Ensure even coverage from roots to ends.
4. **Leave On:** Cover your hair with a shower cap and leave the mask on for 30-60 minutes.
5. **Rinse and Shampoo:** Rinse thoroughly with lukewarm water and shampoo to remove the mask.

5. Hot Oil Treatment

Method Overview:

- **Hot Oil Treatment:** A hot oil treatment with castor oil provides intense hydration and helps repair damaged hair.

Steps:

1. **Prepare the Oil:** Pour a small amount of castor oil into a heat-safe bowl.
2. **Heat the Oil:** Place the bowl in a larger bowl of hot water to warm the oil. Do not microwave the oil, as this can destroy its beneficial properties.
3. **Apply the Oil:** Using your fingertips, apply the warm oil to your scalp and massage gently. Apply the remaining oil to the length of your hair, focusing on the ends.
4. **Wrap and Heat:** Wrap your hair in a warm towel or use a heating cap to maintain warmth. This helps the oil penetrate deeper into the hair shaft.
5. **Leave On:** Leave the oil on for 30-60 minutes.
6. **Rinse and Shampoo:** Rinse thoroughly with lukewarm water and shampoo to remove the oil.

Proper preparation of castor oil enhances its effectiveness and ensures optimal results for your hair care routine. Whether you choose to apply it directly, dilute it with carrier oils, infuse it with essential oils, create a DIY hair mask, or use it as a hot oil treatment, castor oil can provide deep hydration, nourishment, and revitalization for your hair. By following these preparation techniques, you can maximize the benefits of castor oil and achieve healthier, stronger, and more beautiful hair.

Dos and don'ts

Using castor oil effectively in your hair care routine requires knowing the best practices and potential pitfalls. Here are some essential dos and don'ts to ensure you get the most out of castor oil for your hair.

Dos

1. Do Perform a Patch Test

Reason: To ensure you do not have an allergic reaction or sensitivity to castor oil. **How To:**

- **Apply a small amount:** Place a drop of castor oil on a small patch of skin, such as your inner wrist or behind your ear.
- **Wait:** Leave it on for 24 hours and monitor for any signs of redness, itching, or irritation.
- **Assess:** If no reaction occurs, it's safe to use on your scalp and hair.

2. Do Warm the Oil Before Application

Reason: Warm oil penetrates the hair shaft and scalp more effectively. **How To:**

- **Warm it up:** Place the amount of oil you intend to use in a heat-safe bowl and warm it by placing the bowl in a larger bowl of hot water.
- **Avoid microwaving:** Do not microwave the oil, as this can destroy its beneficial properties.

3. Do Massage the Scalp

Reason: Massaging the scalp improves blood circulation, which can promote hair growth. **How To:**

- **Use fingertips:** Use your fingertips to gently massage the oil into your scalp in circular motions.
- **Duration:** Spend 5-10 minutes massaging to ensure even distribution and stimulate the scalp.

4. Do Use a Shower Cap

Reason: A shower cap helps retain heat and enhances oil absorption. **How To:**

- **Cover your hair:** After applying the oil, cover your hair with a shower cap.
- **Leave it on:** Leave the oil on for at least 30 minutes or overnight for a deeper conditioning treatment.

5. Do Rinse Thoroughly

Reason: To remove excess oil and prevent buildup that can weigh hair down. **How To:**

- **Use lukewarm water:** Rinse thoroughly with lukewarm water.
- **Shampoo well:** Use a mild shampoo to remove the oil. You may need to shampoo twice to ensure all the oil is washed out.

6. Do Combine with Other Oils or Ingredients

Reason: Combining castor oil with other beneficial oils or natural ingredients can enhance its effects and make it easier to apply. **How To:**

- **Mix wisely:** Combine castor oil with carrier oils like coconut, jojoba, or argan oil, or with ingredients like honey, yogurt, and eggs for DIY hair masks.

Don'ts

1. Don't Apply Too Much Oil

Reason: Using too much oil can make hair excessively greasy and difficult to wash out. **Avoid:**

- **Excessive application:** Start with a small amount and add more if necessary. A little goes a long way.

2. Don't Leave Oil on Scalp for Too Long

Reason: Leaving oil on for too long, especially overnight, can clog hair follicles and cause scalp issues. **Avoid:**

- **Excessive time:** Limit oil treatments to a few hours or overnight if necessary, but avoid leaving it on for multiple days.

3. Don't Use Castor Oil on Irritated or Broken Skin

Reason: Applying castor oil to irritated or broken skin can exacerbate the condition. **Avoid:**

- **Sensitive areas:** Only use on healthy scalp and hair. If you have scalp issues, consult with a dermatologist before using castor oil.

4. Don't Use Castor Oil Daily

Reason: Daily use can lead to oil buildup and greasy hair. **Avoid:**

- **Overuse:** Limit castor oil treatments to 2-3 times a week for best results without causing buildup.

5. Don't Mix with Harsh Chemicals

Reason: Mixing castor oil with harsh chemicals can reduce its effectiveness and potentially harm your hair. **Avoid:**

- **Chemical mixtures:** Stick to natural ingredients and avoid mixing castor oil with chemical-based hair products.

6. Don't Skip the Patch Test

Reason: Skipping the patch test can lead to unexpected allergic reactions or sensitivities. **Avoid:**

- **Ignoring safety:** Always perform a patch test before using castor oil extensively on your scalp and hair.

Techniques for Applying Castor Oil

Effective application methods

Using castor oil effectively for hair care involves knowing the best application techniques. Proper application ensures that the oil penetrates the hair and scalp, providing maximum benefits. Here are several effective methods for applying castor oil to achieve optimal results.

1. Scalp Massage

Purpose: To stimulate blood circulation, enhance nutrient absorption, and promote hair growth.

Steps:

1. **Warm the Oil:** Pour a small amount of castor oil into a bowl and warm it slightly by placing the bowl in a larger bowl of hot water. Warm oil penetrates better and is more soothing.
2. **Part Your Hair:** Use a comb to part your hair into sections. This ensures even distribution and easier access to the scalp.
3. **Apply to Scalp:** Using your fingertips, apply the warm castor oil directly to your scalp. Start at the roots and work your way around the entire scalp.
4. **Massage Gently:** Massage the oil into your scalp using circular motions. Spend 5-10 minutes massaging to stimulate blood flow and ensure the oil is evenly distributed.
5. **Leave On:** Cover your hair with a shower cap and leave the oil on for at least 30 minutes or overnight for deeper conditioning.
6. **Rinse and Shampoo:** Rinse thoroughly with lukewarm water and shampoo as usual to remove the oil.

2. Hot Oil Treatment

Purpose: To provide intense hydration and repair damaged hair.

Steps:

1. **Prepare the Oil:** Pour a small amount of castor oil into a heat-safe bowl.
2. **Heat the Oil:** Warm the oil by placing the bowl in a larger bowl of hot water. Avoid microwaving to preserve the oil's beneficial properties.
3. **Apply to Hair and Scalp:** Using your fingertips, apply the warm oil to your scalp and massage gently. Apply the remaining oil to the length of your hair, focusing on the ends.
4. **Cover with a Towel:** Wrap your hair in a warm towel or use a heating cap to maintain warmth. This helps the oil penetrate deeper into the hair shaft.
5. **Leave On:** Leave the oil on for 30-60 minutes.
6. **Rinse and Shampoo:** Rinse thoroughly with lukewarm water and shampoo to remove the oil.

3. Overnight Treatment

Purpose: To allow the oil to penetrate deeply and provide maximum nourishment.

Steps:

1. **Warm the Oil:** Pour a small amount of castor oil into a bowl and warm it slightly.
2. **Apply to Scalp and Hair:** Using your fingertips, apply the warm oil to your scalp and massage gently. Apply the remaining oil to the length of your hair.
3. **Cover with a Shower Cap:** Cover your hair with a shower cap to prevent the oil from transferring to your pillow.
4. **Leave On Overnight:** Leave the oil on overnight to allow for deep penetration and maximum benefit.
5. **Rinse and Shampoo:** In the morning, rinse thoroughly with lukewarm water and shampoo to remove the oil.

4. Hair Mask

Purpose: To provide deep conditioning and address specific hair concerns.

Steps:

1. **Gather Ingredients:** Prepare additional ingredients such as honey, yogurt, and egg to combine with castor oil.
2. **Mix the Ingredients:** In a bowl, mix 2 tablespoons of castor oil with 1 tablespoon of honey, 2 tablespoons of yogurt, and 1 egg. Whisk until well combined.
3. **Apply the Mask:** Using your fingertips or a brush, apply the hair mask to your scalp and hair. Ensure even coverage from roots to ends.
4. **Cover and Leave On:** Cover your hair with a shower cap and leave the mask on for 30-60 minutes.
5. **Rinse and Shampoo:** Rinse thoroughly with lukewarm water and shampoo to remove the mask.

5. Pre-Shampoo Treatment

Purpose: To protect hair from the drying effects of shampoo and provide an initial layer of hydration.

Steps:

1. **Apply the Oil:** Before shampooing, apply castor oil to your dry hair and scalp. Focus on the ends and any particularly dry areas.
2. **Leave On:** Leave the oil on for 15-20 minutes.
3. **Shampoo and Condition:** Rinse thoroughly with lukewarm water and shampoo as usual. Follow with your regular conditioner.

6. DIY Hair Serum

Purpose: To provide a lightweight, leave-in treatment for added shine and frizz control.

Steps:

1. **Mix the Oils:** In a small bottle, mix 1 part castor oil with 2 parts lighter carrier oil such as argan or jojoba oil. Add a few drops of essential oils if desired.
2. **Apply Sparingly:** Apply a small amount of the serum to your palms and rub them together. Lightly apply the serum to the ends of your hair and any frizzy areas.
3. **Style as Usual:** Style your hair as usual. This serum can be used on damp or dry hair.

Tips for best results

To maximize the benefits of castor oil for hair care, it's essential to follow best practices and incorporate some expert tips into your routine. These tips will help you achieve healthier, stronger, and more vibrant hair. Here are some valuable tips for getting the best results from using castor oil.

1. Consistency is Key

Regular Application:

- **Frequency:** For optimal results, apply castor oil regularly. Aim for 2-3 times per week.
- **Routine:** Establish a consistent hair care routine to ensure you reap the long-term benefits of castor oil.

2. Combine with Other Oils

Enhance Benefits:

- **Carrier Oils:** Mix castor oil with carrier oils such as coconut oil, jojoba oil, or argan oil. These oils can enhance the moisturizing and nourishing properties of castor oil.
- **Essential Oils:** Add a few drops of essential oils like rosemary, lavender, or peppermint to boost hair growth, soothe the scalp, and add a pleasant scent.

3. Warm the Oil Before Application

Better Absorption:

- **Warmth:** Warming castor oil slightly before application helps it penetrate the hair shaft and scalp more effectively.
- **Method:** Place the oil in a heat-safe bowl and warm it by placing the bowl in a larger bowl of hot water. Avoid using a microwave, as it can destroy beneficial properties.

4. Massage the Scalp

Stimulate Circulation:

- **Massage Technique:** Use your fingertips to massage the oil into your scalp in circular motions. This stimulates blood circulation and enhances nutrient absorption.
- **Duration:** Spend 5-10 minutes massaging the oil into your scalp to ensure even distribution and stimulate hair growth.

5. Use a Shower Cap

Retain Heat:

- **Cover Hair:** After applying castor oil, cover your hair with a shower cap to retain heat and enhance oil absorption.
- **Leave On:** Leave the oil on for at least 30 minutes or overnight for deeper conditioning.

6. Rinse Thoroughly

Prevent Buildup:

- **Rinse Method:** Rinse your hair thoroughly with lukewarm water to remove excess oil. Follow with a mild shampoo to ensure all the oil is washed out.
- **Double Shampoo:** You may need to shampoo twice to remove all traces of oil, especially if you've used a generous amount.

7. Combine with Hair Masks

Deep Conditioning:

- **DIY Masks:** Incorporate castor oil into DIY hair masks with ingredients like honey, yogurt, and eggs for additional hydration and nourishment.
- **Application:** Apply the mask to your hair and scalp, cover with a shower cap, and leave on for 30-60 minutes before rinsing and shampooing.

8. Protect Your Pillow

Overnight Treatments:

- **Pillow Protection:** If you're leaving the oil on overnight, cover your pillow with a towel or use a pillowcase you don't mind getting oily to prevent staining.

9. Use a Clarifying Shampoo

Prevent Oil Buildup:

- **Clarifying:** Occasionally use a clarifying shampoo to remove any buildup of castor oil and other products from your hair.

- **Frequency:** Use a clarifying shampoo once a month to maintain a healthy scalp and hair.

10. Monitor Scalp Health

Avoid Irritation:

- **Patch Test:** Always perform a patch test before using castor oil extensively to ensure you do not have an allergic reaction or sensitivity.
- **Observe:** Monitor your scalp health regularly. If you experience any irritation, redness, or discomfort, reduce the frequency of use or discontinue use.

11. Tailor to Hair Type

Custom Application:

- **Hair Type:** Adjust the amount and frequency of castor oil based on your hair type. Fine hair may require less oil and less frequent application, while thick or coarse hair may benefit from more generous use.
- **Customization:** Experiment with different mixtures and application methods to find what works best for your specific hair type and concerns.

Frequency and Dosage Recommendations

Optimal usage guidelines

To achieve the best results from using castor oil for hair care, it's important to follow optimal usage guidelines. Proper frequency and dosage ensure that your hair receives the right amount of nourishment without causing buildup or other issues. Here, we outline recommended usage frequencies and dosages for various hair concerns and types.

1. General Hair Health and Maintenance

Frequency:

- **Once a Week:** For maintaining healthy hair, applying castor oil once a week is usually sufficient. This regular application helps keep the hair moisturized, strong, and shiny.

Dosage:

- **Amount:** Use about 1-2 tablespoons of castor oil. The exact amount may vary depending on hair length and thickness.
- **Application:** Focus on the scalp and roots, then work the remaining oil through the length of your hair.

2. Dry and Brittle Hair

Frequency:

- **2-3 Times a Week:** For dry and brittle hair, apply castor oil 2-3 times a week to provide intense hydration and restore moisture balance.

Dosage:

- **Amount:** Use 2-3 tablespoons of castor oil. Adjust the quantity based on your hair's dryness and length.
- **Application:** Ensure thorough coverage from scalp to ends. Consider using additional moisturizing agents like coconut oil or honey.

3. Hair Growth and Thickness

Frequency:

- **2-3 Times a Week:** To promote hair growth and increase thickness, apply castor oil 2-3 times a week. Regular application stimulates hair follicles and improves blood circulation to the scalp.

Dosage:

- **Amount:** Use about 2 tablespoons of castor oil.
- **Application:** Massage into the scalp for 5-10 minutes to stimulate blood flow. Cover with a shower cap and leave on for at least 30 minutes or overnight.

4. Scalp Conditions (Dandruff, Seborrheic Dermatitis, Psoriasis)

Frequency:

- **2-3 Times a Week:** For treating scalp conditions, apply castor oil 2-3 times a week to help soothe irritation, reduce inflammation, and control dandruff.

Dosage:

- **Amount:** Use 1-2 tablespoons of castor oil.
- **Application:** Focus on affected areas of the scalp. Massage gently to avoid further irritation. Leave on for at least 30 minutes before rinsing.

5. Damaged Hair

Frequency:

- **Once a Week:** Apply castor oil once a week to repair and strengthen damaged hair. Regular use helps restore hair health and prevent further damage.

Dosage:

- **Amount:** Use 2-3 tablespoons of castor oil, depending on the extent of the damage and hair length.
- **Application:** Focus on the ends and damaged areas. Combine with other nourishing ingredients like yogurt or eggs for a deep conditioning treatment.

6. Oily Scalp and Hair

Frequency:

- **Once a Week:** For oily scalp and hair, apply castor oil once a week. Use a lighter application to avoid excess greasiness.

Dosage:

- **Amount:** Use 1 tablespoon of castor oil mixed with a lighter carrier oil like jojoba oil.
- **Application:** Apply sparingly to the scalp and roots. Avoid heavy application to prevent oil buildup.

7. Fine or Thin Hair

Frequency:

- **Once a Week:** Apply castor oil once a week for fine or thin hair to avoid weighing it down while still providing nourishment.

Dosage:

- **Amount:** Use 1-2 tablespoons of castor oil, possibly mixed with a lighter oil like argan or grapeseed oil.
- **Application:** Apply lightly to the scalp and hair, focusing on areas needing extra care without overloading the hair with oil.

8. Overnight Treatments

Frequency:

- **Once a Week:** Overnight treatments should be done once a week to allow deep penetration and maximum benefits without causing buildup.

Dosage:

- **Amount:** Use 2-3 tablespoons of castor oil, depending on hair length and thickness.
- **Application:** Apply generously to the scalp and hair. Cover with a shower cap and leave on overnight. Wash thoroughly in the morning.

Castor Oil Hair Treatments

Scalp Massage Techniques

Detailed techniques for massages

Scalp massages are a vital part of using castor oil effectively for hair care. They help improve blood circulation, stimulate hair follicles, and enhance nutrient absorption. Here are detailed techniques for performing effective scalp massages with castor oil.

1. Basic Scalp Massage

Purpose: To stimulate blood flow and enhance the absorption of castor oil into the scalp.

Steps:

1. **Warm the Oil:** Pour a small amount of castor oil into a bowl and warm it slightly by placing the bowl in a larger bowl of hot water.
2. **Part Your Hair:** Use a comb to part your hair into sections. This helps ensure the oil reaches the scalp evenly.
3. **Apply the Oil:** Dip your fingertips into the warm oil and apply it directly to your scalp. Start at the front and work your way back.
4. **Use Circular Motions:** Using gentle, circular motions, massage the oil into your scalp. Focus on one section at a time, ensuring even distribution.
5. **Duration:** Spend 5-10 minutes massaging the oil into your scalp. This helps stimulate blood flow and relaxes the scalp muscles.
6. **Cover and Leave On:** Cover your hair with a shower cap and leave the oil on for at least 30 minutes or overnight for deeper conditioning.
7. **Rinse and Shampoo:** Rinse thoroughly with lukewarm water and shampoo as usual to remove the oil.

2. Pressure Point Massage

Purpose: To relieve tension, reduce stress, and promote hair growth by stimulating specific pressure points on the scalp.

Steps:

1. **Warm the Oil:** As with the basic scalp massage, warm the castor oil slightly before application.
2. **Apply to Scalp:** Apply the warm oil to your scalp using your fingertips.
3. **Identify Pressure Points:** Focus on key pressure points such as the temples, the crown of the head, and the base of the skull.
4. **Apply Gentle Pressure:** Use your fingertips to apply gentle pressure to these points. Hold the pressure for a few seconds before moving to the next point.
5. **Circular Motions:** After applying pressure, use circular motions to massage the oil into these areas.
6. **Duration:** Spend about 10-15 minutes focusing on these pressure points.

7. **Cover and Leave On:** Cover your hair with a shower cap and leave the oil on for at least 30 minutes or overnight.
8. **Rinse and Shampoo:** Rinse thoroughly and shampoo to remove the oil.

3. Fingertip Tapping Massage

Purpose: To invigorate the scalp and improve blood circulation using a light, tapping motion.

Steps:

1. **Warm the Oil:** Warm the castor oil slightly before application.
2. **Apply to Scalp:** Apply the warm oil to your scalp using your fingertips.
3. **Light Tapping:** Using your fingertips, gently tap all over your scalp. Start at the forehead and work your way towards the back of your head.
4. **Rhythmic Motion:** Maintain a rhythmic tapping motion to stimulate the scalp without causing irritation.
5. **Combination Technique:** Combine tapping with light circular motions to enhance the massage.
6. **Duration:** Perform the tapping massage for about 5-7 minutes.
7. **Cover and Leave On:** Cover your hair with a shower cap and leave the oil on for at least 30 minutes or overnight.
8. **Rinse and Shampoo:** Rinse thoroughly with lukewarm water and shampoo as usual.

4. Inversion Method

Purpose: To boost hair growth by increasing blood flow to the scalp through inversion.

Steps:

1. **Warm the Oil:** Warm the castor oil slightly before application.
2. **Apply to Scalp:** Apply the warm oil to your scalp using your fingertips.
3. **Massage the Scalp:** Use circular motions to massage the oil into your scalp for 5-10 minutes.
4. **Inversion:** Sit on a chair or bed and lower your head so that it is below your heart level. This position helps increase blood flow to the scalp.
5. **Duration:** Remain in the inverted position for 4-5 minutes. Avoid staying inverted for too long to prevent dizziness.
6. **Return to Upright:** Slowly return to an upright position to avoid a sudden rush of blood.
7. **Cover and Leave On:** Cover your hair with a shower cap and leave the oil on for at least 30 minutes or overnight.
8. **Rinse and Shampoo:** Rinse thoroughly with lukewarm water and shampoo to remove the oil.

5. Combination Massage

Purpose: To combine various techniques for a comprehensive scalp massage that maximizes the benefits of castor oil.

Steps:

1. **Warm the Oil:** Warm the castor oil slightly before application.
2. **Apply to Scalp:** Apply the warm oil to your scalp using your fingertips.
3. **Circular Motions:** Start with gentle circular motions to evenly distribute the oil.
4. **Pressure Points:** Move on to applying gentle pressure to key points on your scalp.
5. **Tapping:** Incorporate light fingertip tapping to invigorate the scalp.
6. **Inversion (Optional):** If comfortable, use the inversion method for a few minutes to enhance blood flow.
7. **Duration:** Spend 10-15 minutes on the massage, combining all techniques.
8. **Cover and Leave On:** Cover your hair with a shower cap and leave the oil on for at least 30 minutes or overnight.
9. **Rinse and Shampoo:** Rinse thoroughly and shampoo as usual.

Incorporating scalp massage techniques into your hair care routine can significantly enhance the benefits of castor oil. Whether you choose the basic scalp massage, pressure point massage, fingertip tapping, inversion method, or a combination of techniques, regular massages can stimulate hair growth, improve scalp health, and ensure better absorption of the oil. By following these detailed techniques, you can achieve healthier, stronger, and more vibrant hair.

Benefits for hair growth

Castor oil is renowned for its remarkable ability to promote hair growth. Its unique composition of nutrients, fatty acids, and vitamins makes it an effective natural remedy for improving hair health and stimulating growth. Here, we explore the detailed benefits of castor oil for hair growth and how it helps achieve thicker, longer, and healthier hair.

1. Stimulates Hair Follicles

Mechanism:

- **Ricinoleic Acid:** Castor oil contains a high concentration of ricinoleic acid, a monounsaturated fatty acid that has been shown to increase blood circulation to the scalp.
- **Increased Blood Flow:** Improved blood circulation ensures that hair follicles receive essential nutrients and oxygen, which are vital for healthy hair growth.

Benefits:

- **Enhanced Follicle Health:** By stimulating hair follicles, castor oil promotes the growth of new hair and supports the health of existing hair.

- **Thicker Hair:** Regular use can lead to thicker and denser hair growth.

2. Anti-Inflammatory Properties

Mechanism:

- **Soothes Scalp:** The anti-inflammatory properties of ricinoleic acid help soothe scalp irritation and reduce inflammation.
- **Healthy Scalp Environment:** A healthy, inflammation-free scalp is crucial for optimal hair growth.

Benefits:

- **Reduced Hair Loss:** Reducing scalp inflammation helps prevent hair loss caused by conditions like dandruff and seborrheic dermatitis.
- **Improved Hair Growth:** A calm and healthy scalp environment fosters better hair growth.

3. Antimicrobial Action

Mechanism:

- **Antibacterial and Antifungal:** Castor oil has natural antibacterial and antifungal properties that help prevent and treat scalp infections.
- **Prevents Scalp Issues:** Conditions such as dandruff, folliculitis, and other scalp infections can impede hair growth.

Benefits:

- **Healthy Scalp:** Keeping the scalp free from infections ensures a healthier environment for hair growth.
- **Stronger Hair:** Healthy scalp conditions lead to stronger hair growth and reduced breakage.

4. Moisturizing and Conditioning

Mechanism:

- **Hydration:** Castor oil is a natural humectant, meaning it attracts and retains moisture in the hair and scalp.
- **Deep Conditioning:** Provides deep conditioning, keeping hair hydrated and preventing dryness and brittleness.

Benefits:

- **Elasticity and Strength:** Well-moisturized hair is more elastic and less prone to breakage.
- **Smooth and Soft Hair:** Hydrated hair is smoother, softer, and more manageable.

5. Rich in Nutrients

Mechanism:

- **Essential Fatty Acids:** Castor oil is rich in essential fatty acids, including omega-6 and omega-9 fatty acids, which are crucial for hair health.
- **Vitamins and Minerals:** Contains vitamin E and other nutrients that nourish the scalp and hair follicles.

Benefits:

- **Nourished Hair:** Provides essential nutrients that support healthy hair growth and repair damage.
- **Stronger Hair:** Nutrient-rich castor oil helps strengthen hair from the roots to the tips.

6. Balances Scalp pH

Mechanism:

- **pH Regulation:** Castor oil helps balance the pH level of the scalp, preventing conditions such as dryness and excessive oiliness.
- **Sebum Regulation:** Regulates the production of sebum, the scalp's natural oil.

Benefits:

- **Healthy Scalp Balance:** A balanced scalp environment supports healthy hair growth and prevents scalp issues.
- **Reduced Scalp Problems:** Maintaining a proper pH level reduces the likelihood of scalp conditions that can hinder hair growth.

7. Prevents Hair Damage

Mechanism:

- **Protective Barrier:** Castor oil forms a protective barrier on the hair shaft, shielding it from environmental damage and chemical treatments.
- **Reduces Protein Loss:** Helps reduce protein loss from hair, which is essential for maintaining hair strength.

Benefits:

- **Damage Protection:** Protects hair from damage caused by environmental factors, heat styling, and chemical treatments.
- **Stronger, Healthier Hair:** Reducing damage and protein loss results in stronger and healthier hair.

8. Prolongs Hair Growth Phase

Mechanism:

- **Anagen Phase Extension:** Castor oil helps prolong the anagen (growth) phase of the hair cycle, allowing hair to grow longer before it enters the resting phase.
- **Improved Hair Cycle:** Supports a healthy hair growth cycle by promoting continuous hair growth.

Benefits:

- **Longer Hair:** Prolonging the growth phase allows hair to reach greater lengths.
- **Fuller Hair:** A longer anagen phase contributes to fuller and denser hair.

Overnight Treatments

How to use castor oil overnight

Overnight treatments with castor oil are an excellent way to deeply condition your hair and scalp, providing ample time for the oil to penetrate and nourish. This method is particularly beneficial for those with dry, damaged, or brittle hair. Here's a detailed guide on how to effectively use castor oil overnight.

1. Preparing for the Treatment

Gather Supplies:

- **Castor Oil:** Use a high-quality, cold-pressed, organic castor oil for the best results.
- **Shower Cap:** A shower cap will keep the oil contained and prevent it from staining your bedding.
- **Old Towel or Pillowcase:** Protect your pillow with an old towel or a pillowcase you don't mind getting oily.

Steps:

1. **Warm the Oil:** Pour a small amount of castor oil into a heat-safe bowl and warm it slightly by placing the bowl in a larger bowl of hot water. Warm oil penetrates the hair and scalp more effectively.
2. **Part Your Hair:** Use a comb to part your hair into sections. This helps ensure the oil reaches the scalp and is evenly distributed.

2. Applying the Oil

Steps:

1. **Apply to Scalp:** Dip your fingertips into the warm castor oil and apply it directly to your scalp. Start at the roots and work your way around the entire scalp.

2. **Massage:** Using gentle, circular motions, massage the oil into your scalp for 5-10 minutes. This stimulates blood circulation and helps the oil absorb better.
3. **Apply to Hair:** Once your scalp is covered, apply the remaining oil to the length of your hair, focusing on the ends, which are usually the most damaged.

3. Covering Your Hair

Steps:

1. **Shower Cap:** After applying the oil, cover your hair with a shower cap. This keeps the oil contained and creates a warm environment that helps the oil penetrate deeply.
2. **Protect Your Pillow:** Place an old towel or a protective pillowcase on your pillow to prevent oil stains.

4. Overnight Rest

Steps:

1. **Sleep with the Oil:** Leave the castor oil on your hair and scalp overnight. This extended period allows the oil to deeply condition and nourish your hair.
2. **Avoid Movement:** Try to sleep in a position that minimizes movement to keep the shower cap in place and prevent leaks.

5. Washing Out the Oil

Steps:

1. **Morning Rinse:** In the morning, start by rinsing your hair with lukewarm water to remove the excess oil.
2. **Shampoo Thoroughly:** Apply a generous amount of shampoo to your hair. You may need to shampoo twice to ensure all the oil is removed. Use a mild or clarifying shampoo for best results.
3. **Condition:** Follow with your regular conditioner to add extra moisture and ensure your hair remains soft and manageable.

6. Frequency of Overnight Treatments

Guidelines:

1. **For Dry and Damaged Hair:** Use overnight treatments 2-3 times a week until your hair shows signs of improvement.
2. **For Maintenance:** Once your hair health improves, reduce the frequency to once a week for maintenance.

7. Additional Tips

Enhance the Treatment:

1. **Add Essential Oils:** Mix a few drops of essential oils like lavender, rosemary, or peppermint into the castor oil for added benefits and a pleasant scent.
2. **Combine with Other Oils:** Blend castor oil with lighter oils such as coconut oil, jojoba oil, or argan oil to enhance its properties and make it easier to apply.

Protect Your Skin:

1. **Avoid Forehead Breakouts:** Be mindful of the oil spreading onto your forehead or face, as it may cause breakouts. Wipe away any excess oil around your hairline before sleeping.

Monitor Scalp Health:

1. **Patch Test:** Always perform a patch test before using castor oil extensively to ensure you do not have an allergic reaction or sensitivity.
2. **Adjust Frequency:** Monitor how your scalp and hair respond to the treatment and adjust the frequency accordingly.

Expected results

Using castor oil as part of your hair care routine can lead to a variety of positive outcomes. While results can vary depending on individual hair type and condition, most people will notice significant improvements in their hair's health, appearance, and growth over time. Here's an in-depth look at the expected results from regular use of castor oil.

1. Improved Hair Growth

Timeline: 1-3 Months

- **Increased Length:** Many users notice increased hair length within a few months of regular application. Castor oil's ability to stimulate hair follicles and improve blood circulation to the scalp contributes to faster hair growth.
- **Fuller Hair:** As new hair growth is stimulated, hair density often improves, resulting in fuller and thicker hair.

2. Enhanced Hair Thickness

Timeline: 2-4 Weeks

- **Stronger Strands:** Castor oil strengthens hair from the roots to the tips, reducing breakage and hair loss. This leads to visibly thicker hair strands.
- **Increased Volume:** Over time, consistent use can increase hair volume, making hair appear fuller and more robust.

3. Reduced Hair Loss

Timeline: 1-2 Months

- **Less Shedding:** Regular scalp massages with castor oil can reduce hair shedding by strengthening hair follicles and reducing scalp inflammation.
- **Healthier Scalp:** A healthier scalp environment helps minimize conditions that cause hair loss, such as dandruff and seborrheic dermatitis.

4. Improved Scalp Health

Timeline: 2-4 Weeks

- **Hydrated Scalp:** Castor oil's moisturizing properties help keep the scalp hydrated, reducing dryness and flakiness.
- **Reduced Dandruff:** Its antifungal and antibacterial properties can help control dandruff and other scalp infections, leading to a healthier scalp.

5. Increased Hair Shine

Timeline: Immediate to 1 Week

- **Natural Luster:** The fatty acids and vitamin E in castor oil add a natural shine to the hair, making it look healthier and more vibrant.
- **Smooth and Silky Texture:** Regular use of castor oil can smooth the hair cuticle, resulting in a silky and shiny appearance.

6. Enhanced Hair Manageability

Timeline: 2-4 Weeks

- **Easier Styling:** Castor oil helps detangle hair, making it easier to comb and style. This is particularly beneficial for curly and coily hair types.
- **Less Frizz:** Its moisturizing properties reduce frizz and flyaways, leading to smoother, more manageable hair.

7. Repair of Damaged Hair

Timeline: 1-3 Months

- **Reduced Split Ends:** Castor oil helps repair and seal split ends, preventing further damage and promoting healthier hair growth.
- **Stronger Hair:** The strengthening properties of castor oil help repair damage caused by heat styling, chemical treatments, and environmental factors.

8. Balanced Scalp Oil Production

Timeline: 2-4 Weeks

- **Normalized Sebum Production:** Castor oil helps balance the scalp's natural oil production, reducing excessive oiliness or dryness.
- **Healthy Scalp Environment:** A balanced scalp pH and regulated sebum production contribute to overall scalp health and optimal hair growth conditions.

9. Long-Term Benefits

Timeline: 6 Months and Beyond

- **Sustained Hair Health:** Continued use of castor oil can lead to long-term improvements in hair health, including stronger, thicker, and more resilient hair.
- **Prevention of Future Damage:** Regular application can help protect hair from future damage by maintaining moisture levels and strengthening the hair shaft.

Hot Oil Treatments

Procedure for hot oil treatment

Hot oil treatments are a luxurious and effective way to nourish and revitalize your hair. Using castor oil for a hot oil treatment can deeply condition your hair, improve its strength, and enhance its overall health. Here's a step-by-step guide to performing a hot oil treatment with castor oil.

1. Gather Your Supplies

Essentials:

- **Castor Oil:** Choose a high-quality, cold-pressed, organic castor oil for the best results.
- **Carrier Oil:** Consider blending with lighter oils like coconut oil, jojoba oil, or olive oil for added benefits and easier application.
- **Essential Oils:** Optional, but beneficial. Essential oils like rosemary, lavender, or peppermint can enhance the treatment.
- **Heat-Safe Bowl:** For warming the oil.
- **Shower Cap:** To retain heat and protect your surroundings.
- **Towel:** To wrap around your head and keep the oil warm.

2. Prepare the Oil

Steps:

1. **Measure the Oil:** Pour 2-3 tablespoons of castor oil into a heat-safe bowl. Adjust the amount based on your hair length and thickness.
2. **Add Carrier Oil:** Mix in equal parts of a carrier oil if desired. This makes the oil easier to apply and adds additional nutrients.
3. **Essential Oils:** Add a few drops of essential oil for added benefits and a pleasant aroma.

3. Heat the Oil

Steps:

1. **Warm the Oil:** Place the bowl with the oil mixture into a larger bowl filled with hot water. Let it sit for a few minutes until the oil is warm. Ensure the oil is warm but not hot to avoid burning your scalp.
2. **Test the Temperature:** Dip your fingertip into the oil to check the temperature. It should be comfortably warm.

4. Prepare Your Hair

Steps:

1. **Detangle Hair:** Gently comb your hair to remove any tangles. This helps with even application.
2. **Section Your Hair:** Divide your hair into manageable sections using hair clips. This ensures the oil reaches every part of your scalp and hair.

5. Apply the Oil

Steps:

1. **Scalp Application:** Dip your fingertips into the warm oil and apply it directly to your scalp. Massage gently in circular motions to stimulate blood circulation.
2. **Hair Application:** Apply the remaining oil to the length of your hair, focusing on the ends, which are often the most damaged.
3. **Even Distribution:** Ensure the oil is evenly distributed by combing through your hair with a wide-tooth comb.

6. Massage Your Scalp

Steps:

1. **Circular Motions:** Use your fingertips to massage your scalp in circular motions for 5-10 minutes. This enhances blood flow and helps the oil penetrate deeply.
2. **Pressure Points:** Focus on pressure points like the temples, crown, and base of the skull for added relaxation and stimulation.

7. Cover Your Hair

Steps:

1. **Shower Cap:** Cover your hair with a shower cap to retain heat and prevent the oil from dripping.
2. **Towel Wrap:** Wrap a warm towel around your head over the shower cap to maintain the warmth. You can heat the towel in a dryer or dip it in hot water and wring it out before wrapping.

8. Let the Oil Sit

Steps:

1. **Duration:** Leave the oil on your hair for at least 30 minutes. For deeper conditioning, you can leave it on for up to an hour.
2. **Relax:** Use this time to relax. Read a book, watch a movie, or enjoy a moment of quiet.

9. Rinse and Shampoo

Steps:

1. **Rinse Thoroughly:** Rinse your hair thoroughly with lukewarm water to remove the excess oil.
2. **Shampoo:** Apply a generous amount of shampoo to your hair. You may need to shampoo twice to ensure all the oil is washed out.
3. **Condition:** Follow with your regular conditioner to add extra moisture and ensure your hair remains soft and manageable.

10. Dry and Style

Steps:

1. **Towel Dry:** Gently towel-dry your hair to remove excess water.
2. **Air Dry or Blow Dry:** Let your hair air dry or blow dry it on a low heat setting.
3. **Style:** Style your hair as usual. You'll notice your hair feels softer, shinier, and more manageable.

11. Frequency of Hot Oil Treatments

Guidelines:

1. **Dry and Damaged Hair:** Perform a hot oil treatment once a week to restore moisture and repair damage.
2. **Oily or Fine Hair:** Limit to once every two weeks to avoid excessive oil buildup.
3. **Maintenance:** For general maintenance, a hot oil treatment once a month can keep your hair healthy and strong.

Benefits for hair and scalp

Castor oil is a versatile and powerful natural remedy for various hair and scalp issues. Its unique properties and rich nutrient profile make it highly effective in promoting overall hair and scalp health. Here, we explore the detailed benefits of castor oil for both hair and scalp.

1. Promotes Hair Growth

Mechanism:

- **Ricinoleic Acid:** Castor oil contains a high concentration of ricinoleic acid, which improves blood circulation to the scalp, stimulating hair follicles and promoting growth.
- **Nutrient Delivery:** Enhanced blood flow ensures that hair follicles receive essential nutrients and oxygen.

Benefits:

- **Increased Length:** Regular use can result in longer hair due to stimulated hair growth.
- **Fuller Hair:** Leads to thicker and denser hair as new hair growth is encouraged.

2. Strengthens Hair

Mechanism:

- **Protein Retention:** Castor oil helps reduce protein loss from hair, which is crucial for maintaining hair strength.
- **Fatty Acids:** The oil's fatty acids nourish the hair shaft, reinforcing hair structure and reducing breakage.

Benefits:

- **Less Breakage:** Stronger hair is less prone to breakage and split ends.
- **Enhanced Durability:** Hair becomes more resilient to physical and environmental stress.

3. Deep Moisturization

Mechanism:

- **Humectant Properties:** Castor oil is a natural humectant that attracts and retains moisture in the hair and scalp.
- **Deep Penetration:** Penetrates deeply into the hair shaft and scalp, providing long-lasting hydration.

Benefits:

- **Hydrated Hair:** Keeps hair well-moisturized, preventing dryness and brittleness.
- **Smooth Texture:** Results in softer, smoother hair with a healthy shine.

4. Improves Scalp Health

Mechanism:

- **Antimicrobial Action:** Castor oil has natural antibacterial and antifungal properties that help prevent and treat scalp infections.
- **Anti-Inflammatory:** The anti-inflammatory properties of ricinoleic acid soothe scalp irritation and reduce inflammation.

Benefits:

- **Reduced Dandruff:** Helps control dandruff and other scalp conditions by maintaining a healthy scalp environment.
- **Soothed Scalp:** Provides relief from itching and irritation, promoting a healthy scalp.

5. Enhances Hair Thickness

Mechanism:

- **Nutrient Supply:** Rich in essential nutrients, vitamins, and fatty acids that nourish hair follicles.
- **Follicle Stimulation:** Stimulates dormant hair follicles, promoting the growth of new hair.

Benefits:

- **Thicker Hair:** Regular application can result in visibly thicker and more voluminous hair.
- **Increased Density:** Enhances hair density by stimulating new hair growth.

6. Adds Natural Shine

Mechanism:

- **Seals Cuticles:** Castor oil smooths and seals the hair cuticle, reflecting light and adding natural shine.
- **Nutrient-Rich:** The vitamins and fatty acids in castor oil nourish the hair, enhancing its luster.

Benefits:

- **Glossy Hair:** Hair appears shinier and healthier.
- **Smooth Finish:** Provides a smooth and polished look, reducing frizz and flyaways.

7. Repairs Damaged Hair

Mechanism:

- **Deep Conditioning:** Provides intense hydration and nourishment that helps repair damaged hair.
- **Protective Barrier:** Forms a protective layer on the hair shaft, shielding it from environmental damage and chemical treatments.

Benefits:

- **Damage Repair:** Helps repair and restore hair damaged by heat styling, coloring, and environmental exposure.
- **Healthier Hair:** Results in healthier, more resilient hair that is less prone to damage.

8. Balances Scalp Oil Production

Mechanism:

- **Sebum Regulation:** Helps regulate the production of sebum, the scalp's natural oil.
- **pH Balance:** Balances the scalp's pH level, preventing excessive oiliness or dryness.

Benefits:

- **Healthy Scalp Balance:** Maintains a healthy scalp environment, supporting optimal hair growth.
- **Reduced Scalp Issues:** Prevents scalp conditions caused by imbalanced oil production.

9. Soothes Scalp Conditions

Mechanism:

- **Anti-Inflammatory:** Reduces inflammation associated with scalp conditions like psoriasis and seborrheic dermatitis.
- **Moisturizing:** Keeps the scalp moisturized, reducing dryness and flakiness.

Benefits:

- **Relief from Conditions:** Provides relief from conditions such as dandruff, psoriasis, and seborrheic dermatitis.
- **Calm and Healthy Scalp:** Promotes a calm and healthy scalp, which is essential for healthy hair growth.

10. Protects Hair

Mechanism:

- **Barrier Formation:** Forms a protective barrier on the hair shaft, shielding it from environmental pollutants and UV rays.
- **Damage Prevention:** Helps prevent damage from heat styling and chemical treatments.

Benefits:

- **Environmental Protection:** Protects hair from damage caused by environmental factors.
- **Longevity of Hair Health:** Maintains the health and integrity of the hair over time.

Conclusion

Castor oil offers a wide range of benefits for both hair and scalp health. Its ability to promote hair growth, strengthen hair, deeply moisturize, and improve scalp health makes it an invaluable addition to any hair care routine. By incorporating castor oil into your regular hair care regimen, you can achieve healthier, stronger, and more beautiful hair. Regular use can lead to significant improvements in hair texture, thickness, shine, and overall vitality.

DIY Castor Oil Hair Recipes

Hair Masks

Recipes and instructions

DIY hair masks made with castor oil can provide deep conditioning, nourishment, and repair for various hair types and concerns. These recipes combine castor oil with other beneficial ingredients to address specific hair issues. Here are some effective castor oil hair mask recipes and detailed instructions on how to use them.

1. Castor Oil and Honey Hair Mask

Purpose: To deeply moisturize and add shine to dry, dull hair.

Ingredients:

- 2 tablespoons of castor oil
- 1 tablespoon of honey
- 1 egg (optional, for added protein)

Instructions:

1. **Mix Ingredients:** In a bowl, combine 2 tablespoons of castor oil and 1 tablespoon of honey. If desired, add 1 egg for extra protein and whisk until well blended.
2. **Apply to Hair:** Apply the mixture to your scalp and hair, focusing on the ends.
3. **Massage:** Massage gently into the scalp for 5-10 minutes to ensure even distribution and stimulate blood circulation.
4. **Cover and Leave On:** Cover your hair with a shower cap and leave the mask on for 30-60 minutes.
5. **Rinse and Shampoo:** Rinse thoroughly with lukewarm water and shampoo to remove the mask. Follow with conditioner if needed.

Benefits:

- **Moisturizes:** Honey is a natural humectant that helps retain moisture.
- **Adds Shine:** Leaves hair shiny and smooth.
- **Strengthens:** Egg provides protein, strengthening hair and preventing breakage.

2. Castor Oil and Avocado Hair Mask

Purpose: To nourish and repair damaged hair.

Ingredients:

- 2 tablespoons of castor oil
- 1 ripe avocado
- 1 tablespoon of coconut oil

Instructions:

1. **Prepare Avocado:** Mash the ripe avocado in a bowl until smooth.
2. **Mix Ingredients:** Add 2 tablespoons of castor oil and 1 tablespoon of coconut oil to the mashed avocado. Mix thoroughly.
3. **Apply to Hair:** Apply the mixture to your hair, focusing on the ends and any damaged areas.
4. **Massage:** Massage into the scalp and hair for 5-10 minutes.
5. **Cover and Leave On:** Cover your hair with a shower cap and leave the mask on for 30-60 minutes.
6. **Rinse and Shampoo:** Rinse thoroughly with lukewarm water and shampoo to remove the mask. Follow with conditioner if needed.

Benefits:

- **Repairs Damage:** Avocado is rich in vitamins and fatty acids that repair and strengthen hair.
- **Deep Conditioning:** Coconut oil adds extra moisture and smoothness.

3. Castor Oil and Aloe Vera Hair Mask

Purpose: To soothe the scalp and promote hair growth.

Ingredients:

- 2 tablespoons of castor oil
- 2 tablespoons of aloe vera gel
- 1 tablespoon of olive oil

Instructions:

1. **Mix Ingredients:** In a bowl, combine 2 tablespoons of castor oil, 2 tablespoons of aloe vera gel, and 1 tablespoon of olive oil. Mix until well blended.
2. **Apply to Hair:** Apply the mixture to your scalp and hair, focusing on the roots.
3. **Massage:** Massage gently into the scalp for 5-10 minutes to stimulate blood circulation.
4. **Cover and Leave On:** Cover your hair with a shower cap and leave the mask on for 30-60 minutes.
5. **Rinse and Shampoo:** Rinse thoroughly with lukewarm water and shampoo to remove the mask. Follow with conditioner if needed.

Benefits:

- **Soothes Scalp:** Aloe vera has anti-inflammatory properties that soothe the scalp.
- **Promotes Growth:** Stimulates hair follicles and promotes hair growth.

4. Castor Oil and Yogurt Hair Mask

Purpose: To hydrate and soften hair.

Ingredients:

- 2 tablespoons of castor oil
- 2 tablespoons of plain yogurt
- 1 tablespoon of honey

Instructions:

1. **Mix Ingredients:** In a bowl, combine 2 tablespoons of castor oil, 2 tablespoons of plain yogurt, and 1 tablespoon of honey. Mix until smooth.
2. **Apply to Hair:** Apply the mixture to your hair, focusing on the ends and any dry areas.
3. **Massage:** Massage into the scalp and hair for 5-10 minutes.
4. **Cover and Leave On:** Cover your hair with a shower cap and leave the mask on for 30-60 minutes.
5. **Rinse and Shampoo:** Rinse thoroughly with lukewarm water and shampoo to remove the mask. Follow with conditioner if needed.

Benefits:

- **Hydrates:** Yogurt provides deep hydration and smoothness.
- **Softens:** Honey helps to soften and add shine to the hair.

5. Castor Oil and Banana Hair Mask

Purpose: To nourish and strengthen hair.

Ingredients:

- 2 tablespoons of castor oil
- 1 ripe banana
- 1 tablespoon of olive oil

Instructions:

1. **Prepare Banana:** Mash the ripe banana in a bowl until smooth.
2. **Mix Ingredients:** Add 2 tablespoons of castor oil and 1 tablespoon of olive oil to the mashed banana. Mix thoroughly.
3. **Apply to Hair:** Apply the mixture to your hair, focusing on the scalp and ends.
4. **Massage:** Massage into the scalp and hair for 5-10 minutes.
5. **Cover and Leave On:** Cover your hair with a shower cap and leave the mask on for 30-60 minutes.
6. **Rinse and Shampoo:** Rinse thoroughly with lukewarm water and shampoo to remove the mask. Follow with conditioner if needed.

Benefits:

- **Nourishes:** Banana is rich in vitamins and minerals that nourish hair.
- **Strengthens:** Olive oil adds strength and shine to the hair.

DIY castor oil hair masks are an excellent way to provide your hair with deep conditioning, nourishment, and repair. These recipes combine castor oil with other natural ingredients to address specific hair concerns, from dryness and damage to lack of shine and growth. By incorporating these masks into your hair care routine, you can achieve healthier, stronger, and more beautiful hair.

Benefits of each mask

Each DIY castor oil hair mask combines castor oil with other natural ingredients to address specific hair concerns. Here, we expand on the detailed benefits of each mask and how they contribute to healthier, stronger, and more beautiful hair.

1. Castor Oil and Honey Hair Mask

Ingredients:

- 2 tablespoons of castor oil
- 1 tablespoon of honey
- 1 egg (optional, for added protein)

Benefits:

- **Deep Moisturization:** Honey is a natural humectant that attracts and retains moisture. This mask deeply hydrates the hair, making it softer and more manageable.
- **Enhanced Shine:** Honey adds a natural shine to the hair, leaving it looking glossy and healthy.
- **Strengthening:** The egg, rich in proteins, helps strengthen the hair strands, reducing breakage and split ends. Protein treatments are essential for rebuilding and repairing hair structure.
- **Scalp Health:** Castor oil's antimicrobial properties help maintain a healthy scalp, reducing dandruff and preventing scalp infections.

2. Castor Oil and Avocado Hair Mask

Ingredients:

- 2 tablespoons of castor oil
- 1 ripe avocado
- 1 tablespoon of coconut oil

Benefits:

- **Repair and Nourishment:** Avocado is packed with vitamins A, D, E, and B6, as well as folic acid, amino acids, and fatty acids. These nutrients nourish and repair damaged hair, restoring its natural strength and elasticity.

- **Deep Conditioning:** Coconut oil penetrates the hair shaft deeply, providing intense hydration and reducing protein loss.
- **Smooth and Soft Hair:** The combined moisturizing effects of avocado and coconut oil leave hair feeling smooth, soft, and manageable.
- **Reduced Frizz:** This mask helps to tame frizz and flyaways, making hair easier to style.

3. Castor Oil and Aloe Vera Hair Mask

Ingredients:

- 2 tablespoons of castor oil
- 2 tablespoons of aloe vera gel
- 1 tablespoon of olive oil

Benefits:

- **Scalp Soothing:** Aloe vera has anti-inflammatory properties that soothe the scalp, reducing irritation, itching, and redness. It also helps to heal any minor scalp abrasions.
- **Hair Growth Stimulation:** Aloe vera contains proteolytic enzymes that repair dead skin cells on the scalp and stimulate dormant hair follicles, promoting hair growth.
- **Enhanced Moisture:** Olive oil adds moisture to the hair and scalp, preventing dryness and flakiness.
- **Nutrient Delivery:** The vitamins and minerals in aloe vera nourish the hair, improving its overall health and appearance.

4. Castor Oil and Yogurt Hair Mask

Ingredients:

- 2 tablespoons of castor oil
- 2 tablespoons of plain yogurt
- 1 tablespoon of honey

Benefits:

- **Hydration and Softness:** Yogurt contains lactic acid, which helps to hydrate and soften the hair. It also has antibacterial properties that keep the scalp healthy.
- **Shine and Manageability:** Honey adds shine and smoothness, making hair more manageable and easier to style.
- **Scalp Health:** The probiotics in yogurt help maintain a healthy scalp microbiome, reducing the risk of dandruff and other scalp conditions.
- **Strengthening:** This mask strengthens hair strands, reducing breakage and promoting healthier hair growth.

5. Castor Oil and Banana Hair Mask

Ingredients:

- 2 tablespoons of castor oil
- 1 ripe banana
- 1 tablespoon of olive oil

Benefits:

- **Nourishment and Strength:** Bananas are rich in potassium, natural oils, carbohydrates, and vitamins, which help to soften the hair and protect its natural elasticity.
- **Moisture and Shine:** Olive oil deeply moisturizes and adds shine, making hair look and feel healthier.
- **Frizz Control:** This mask helps to control frizz and flyaways, making hair smoother and more manageable.
- **Repair and Protection:** The nutrients in banana and olive oil repair damaged hair and protect it from future damage, including heat and environmental factors.

Conditioners

Homemade conditioner recipes

Creating your own homemade conditioners with castor oil can provide your hair with the nourishment it needs without the use of harsh chemicals found in many commercial products. Here are some effective castor oil-based conditioner recipes and detailed instructions for their use.

1. Castor Oil and Coconut Milk Conditioner

Purpose: To deeply moisturize and strengthen hair.

Ingredients:

- 2 tablespoons of castor oil
- 1/2 cup of coconut milk
- 1 tablespoon of honey

Instructions:

1. **Mix Ingredients:** In a bowl, combine 2 tablespoons of castor oil, 1/2 cup of coconut milk, and 1 tablespoon of honey. Stir until well blended.
2. **Application:** After shampooing, apply the mixture to your hair, focusing on the ends and any particularly dry areas.
3. **Massage:** Gently massage the conditioner into your hair and scalp for a few minutes.

4. **Leave On:** Let the conditioner sit in your hair for 5-10 minutes to allow the ingredients to penetrate.
5. **Rinse:** Rinse thoroughly with lukewarm water. Ensure all the conditioner is washed out to avoid any residue.

Benefits:

- **Deep Hydration:** Coconut milk is rich in vitamins and fatty acids that deeply hydrate the hair.
- **Added Shine:** Honey adds a natural shine, making hair look healthier.
- **Strengthening:** Castor oil strengthens hair, reducing breakage and split ends.

2. Castor Oil and Aloe Vera Conditioner

Purpose: To soothe the scalp and condition hair.

Ingredients:

- 2 tablespoons of castor oil
- 1/4 cup of aloe vera gel
- 1 teaspoon of lemon juice (optional, for added shine)

Instructions:

1. **Mix Ingredients:** In a bowl, combine 2 tablespoons of castor oil, 1/4 cup of aloe vera gel, and 1 teaspoon of lemon juice. Mix until smooth.
2. **Application:** Apply the conditioner to damp hair after shampooing, starting from the scalp and working your way down to the ends.
3. **Massage:** Gently massage into your scalp and hair.
4. **Leave On:** Let the conditioner sit for 5-10 minutes to allow the aloe vera to soothe the scalp and the castor oil to condition the hair.
5. **Rinse:** Rinse thoroughly with lukewarm water.

Benefits:

- **Soothing:** Aloe vera soothes the scalp, reducing inflammation and irritation.
- **Conditioning:** Castor oil conditions and nourishes the hair.
- **Shine:** Lemon juice can add a healthy shine to your hair.

3. Castor Oil and Shea Butter Conditioner

Purpose: To deeply nourish and repair damaged hair.

Ingredients:

- 2 tablespoons of castor oil
- 2 tablespoons of shea butter
- 1 tablespoon of argan oil

Instructions:

1. **Melt Shea Butter:** Melt 2 tablespoons of shea butter in a double boiler or microwave until it becomes a liquid.
2. **Mix Ingredients:** Combine the melted shea butter with 2 tablespoons of castor oil and 1 tablespoon of argan oil. Mix well.
3. **Application:** Apply the conditioner to damp hair after shampooing, focusing on the mid-lengths to the ends.
4. **Massage:** Gently massage into your hair to ensure even distribution.
5. **Leave On:** Let the conditioner sit for 10-15 minutes to allow the shea butter and oils to penetrate deeply.
6. **Rinse:** Rinse thoroughly with lukewarm water to remove all traces of the conditioner.

Benefits:

- **Deep Nourishment:** Shea butter provides deep nourishment, repairing and strengthening damaged hair.
- **Hydration:** Argan oil adds hydration and softness.
- **Protection:** Castor oil helps protect the hair from environmental damage.

4. Castor Oil and Yogurt Conditioner

Purpose: To hydrate and soften hair.

Ingredients:

- 2 tablespoons of castor oil
- 1/4 cup of plain yogurt
- 1 tablespoon of olive oil

Instructions:

1. **Mix Ingredients:** In a bowl, combine 2 tablespoons of castor oil, 1/4 cup of plain yogurt, and 1 tablespoon of olive oil. Stir until well blended.
2. **Application:** Apply the mixture to your hair after shampooing, starting at the scalp and working through to the ends.
3. **Massage:** Gently massage into your scalp and hair for a few minutes.
4. **Leave On:** Allow the conditioner to sit for 5-10 minutes.
5. **Rinse:** Rinse thoroughly with lukewarm water to ensure all the conditioner is removed.

Benefits:

- **Hydration:** Yogurt hydrates and softens the hair.
- **Nourishment:** Olive oil adds extra nourishment and shine.
- **Scalp Health:** The probiotics in yogurt help maintain a healthy scalp.

5. Castor Oil and Egg Conditioner

Purpose: To strengthen and repair weak or damaged hair.

Ingredients:

- 2 tablespoons of castor oil
- 1 egg
- 1 tablespoon of honey

Instructions:

1. **Mix Ingredients:** In a bowl, whisk together 2 tablespoons of castor oil, 1 egg, and 1 tablespoon of honey until well combined.
2. **Application:** Apply the mixture to your hair after shampooing, focusing on the roots and ends.
3. **Massage:** Gently massage the conditioner into your hair and scalp.
4. **Leave On:** Let the conditioner sit for 10-15 minutes.
5. **Rinse:** Rinse thoroughly with lukewarm water. Be sure to rinse well to remove all the egg residue.

Benefits:

- **Strengthening:** Egg provides protein that strengthens hair and reduces breakage.
- **Moisturization:** Honey and castor oil hydrate and moisturize the hair.
- **Repair:** This conditioner helps repair damaged hair, making it smoother and more resilient.

Homemade castor oil conditioners are an excellent way to provide your hair with the nourishment it needs without the use of harsh chemicals. These recipes combine the moisturizing, strengthening, and repairing properties of castor oil with other natural ingredients to address specific hair concerns. By incorporating these conditioners into your regular hair care routine, you can achieve healthier, stronger, and more beautiful hair.

How to use them

Step-by-Step Guide to Using Homemade Castor Oil Conditioners

Using homemade castor oil conditioners effectively involves understanding the best practices for application, timing, and removal. Here's a detailed step-by-step guide on how to use each of these conditioners to maximize their benefits.

1. Castor Oil and Coconut Milk Conditioner

Purpose: To deeply moisturize and strengthen hair.

Application Steps:

1. **Prepare Your Hair:** Begin by shampooing your hair with a mild shampoo to remove any dirt, oil, or product buildup.
2. **Mix the Ingredients:** In a bowl, mix 2 tablespoons of castor oil, 1/2 cup of coconut milk, and 1 tablespoon of honey until well blended.
3. **Apply the Conditioner:** While your hair is still damp, apply the mixture starting from the scalp and working your way to the ends. Ensure even distribution.
4. **Massage the Scalp:** Gently massage your scalp with your fingertips for 3-5 minutes to stimulate blood circulation and ensure the conditioner penetrates.
5. **Leave On:** Cover your hair with a shower cap and leave the conditioner on for 5-10 minutes to allow deep penetration.
6. **Rinse Thoroughly:** Rinse your hair thoroughly with lukewarm water to remove all traces of the conditioner.
7. **Dry and Style:** Towel dry your hair and style as usual.

2. Castor Oil and Aloe Vera Conditioner

Purpose: To soothe the scalp and condition hair.

Application Steps:

1. **Prepare Your Hair:** Shampoo your hair with a gentle shampoo and rinse thoroughly.
2. **Mix the Ingredients:** Combine 2 tablespoons of castor oil, 1/4 cup of aloe vera gel, and 1 teaspoon of lemon juice (optional) in a bowl and mix well.
3. **Apply the Conditioner:** Apply the mixture to your damp hair, starting from the roots and working towards the ends.
4. **Scalp Massage:** Massage the conditioner into your scalp for 3-5 minutes to promote absorption and improve scalp health.
5. **Leave On:** Let the conditioner sit on your hair for 5-10 minutes.
6. **Rinse Thoroughly:** Rinse with lukewarm water, ensuring all the conditioner is washed out.
7. **Dry and Style:** Dry your hair with a towel and style as desired.

3. Castor Oil and Shea Butter Conditioner

Purpose: To deeply nourish and repair damaged hair.

Application Steps:

1. **Prepare Your Hair:** Start by washing your hair with a mild shampoo and rinse well.
2. **Mix the Ingredients:** Melt 2 tablespoons of shea butter and combine it with 2 tablespoons of castor oil and 1 tablespoon of argan oil in a bowl. Mix thoroughly.
3. **Apply the Conditioner:** Apply the mixture to damp hair, focusing on the mid-lengths and ends.
4. **Massage:** Gently massage the conditioner into your hair for 3-5 minutes to ensure even distribution.

5. **Leave On:** Cover your hair with a shower cap and leave the conditioner on for 10-15 minutes.
6. **Rinse Thoroughly:** Rinse with lukewarm water until all the conditioner is removed.
7. **Dry and Style:** Towel dry your hair and style as usual.

4. Castor Oil and Yogurt Conditioner

Purpose: To hydrate and soften hair.

Application Steps:

1. **Prepare Your Hair:** Shampoo your hair with a gentle shampoo and rinse thoroughly.
2. **Mix the Ingredients:** In a bowl, combine 2 tablespoons of castor oil, 1/4 cup of plain yogurt, and 1 tablespoon of olive oil. Mix until smooth.
3. **Apply the Conditioner:** Apply the mixture to your damp hair, starting from the scalp and working through to the ends.
4. **Massage:** Massage the conditioner into your scalp and hair for 3-5 minutes.
5. **Leave On:** Let the conditioner sit on your hair for 5-10 minutes.
6. **Rinse Thoroughly:** Rinse with lukewarm water to ensure all the conditioner is removed.
7. **Dry and Style:** Towel dry your hair and style as desired.

5. Castor Oil and Egg Conditioner

Purpose: To strengthen and repair weak or damaged hair.

Application Steps:

1. **Prepare Your Hair:** Wash your hair with a mild shampoo and rinse thoroughly.
2. **Mix the Ingredients:** In a bowl, whisk together 2 tablespoons of castor oil, 1 egg, and 1 tablespoon of honey until well combined.
3. **Apply the Conditioner:** Apply the mixture to your damp hair, focusing on the roots and ends.
4. **Massage:** Massage the conditioner into your scalp and hair for 3-5 minutes.
5. **Leave On:** Cover your hair with a shower cap and leave the conditioner on for 10-15 minutes.
6. **Rinse Thoroughly:** Rinse with lukewarm water. Ensure you rinse well to remove all egg residue.
7. **Dry and Style:** Towel dry your hair and style as usual.

General Tips for Using Homemade Conditioners:

1. Consistent Use: For best results, use these conditioners regularly. Incorporate them into your weekly hair care routine. **2. Gentle Shampoo:** Always start with a gentle shampoo to cleanse your hair without stripping it of natural oils. **3. Lukewarm Water:** Use lukewarm water for rinsing. Hot water can strip your hair of moisture, while cold water may not effectively remove the conditioner. **4. Towel Dry:** Gently towel dry your hair to avoid breakage. Avoid vigorous rubbing. **5. Avoid Overuse:** While these conditioners are beneficial, using them too frequently can lead to product buildup. Adjust the frequency based on your hair's needs.

Using homemade castor oil conditioners can significantly improve the health and appearance of your hair. By following these detailed application steps, you can maximize the benefits of each conditioner, whether your goal is to moisturize, strengthen, repair, or add shine. Regular use of these natural conditioners can lead to healthier, stronger, and more beautiful hair, free from the harsh chemicals found in many commercial products.

Serums and Sprays

DIY serum and spray formulations

Serums and sprays are great ways to incorporate castor oil into your hair care routine without the heaviness that oils sometimes bring. These lightweight formulations can help address various hair concerns, from frizz control to adding shine and promoting growth. Here are some effective DIY castor oil serum and spray recipes, along with detailed instructions on how to make and use them.

1. Castor Oil Hair Growth Serum

Purpose: To promote hair growth and strengthen hair.

Ingredients:

- 2 tablespoons of castor oil
- 2 tablespoons of jojoba oil
- 10 drops of rosemary essential oil
- 10 drops of peppermint essential oil

Instructions:

1. **Mix Ingredients:** In a small bottle with a dropper, combine 2 tablespoons of castor oil and 2 tablespoons of jojoba oil.
2. **Add Essential Oils:** Add 10 drops of rosemary essential oil and 10 drops of peppermint essential oil to the bottle.
3. **Shake Well:** Shake the bottle well to mix the oils thoroughly.

How to Use:

1. **Apply to Scalp:** Use the dropper to apply a few drops of the serum to your scalp. Part your hair in sections to ensure even application.
2. **Massage:** Gently massage the serum into your scalp using circular motions for 5-10 minutes. This helps stimulate blood flow and promotes absorption.
3. **Leave On:** Leave the serum on overnight or for at least 1-2 hours before washing your hair.

4. **Frequency:** Use the serum 2-3 times a week for best results.

Benefits:

- **Promotes Growth:** Rosemary and peppermint essential oils stimulate hair follicles and promote growth.
- **Strengthens Hair:** Jojoba oil helps strengthen hair and prevent breakage.

2. Castor Oil Anti-Frizz Serum

Purpose: To tame frizz and add shine.

Ingredients:

- 1 tablespoon of castor oil
- 1 tablespoon of argan oil
- 5 drops of lavender essential oil

Instructions:

1. **Mix Ingredients:** In a small bottle with a pump, combine 1 tablespoon of castor oil and 1 tablespoon of argan oil.
2. **Add Essential Oil:** Add 5 drops of lavender essential oil to the bottle.
3. **Shake Well:** Shake the bottle well to mix the oils thoroughly.

How to Use:

1. **Apply to Damp Hair:** After washing your hair, apply a small amount of the serum to your damp hair. Focus on the ends and any frizzy areas.
2. **Distribute Evenly:** Use your fingers or a wide-tooth comb to distribute the serum evenly.
3. **Style as Usual:** Let your hair air dry or style as usual.

Benefits:

- **Tames Frizz:** Castor oil and argan oil work together to smooth the hair cuticle and reduce frizz.
- **Adds Shine:** Lavender essential oil adds a pleasant scent and additional shine.

3. Castor Oil Leave-In Conditioning Spray

Purpose: To hydrate and detangle hair.

Ingredients:

- 1 tablespoon of castor oil
- 2 tablespoons of aloe vera juice
- 1 cup of distilled water
- 10 drops of tea tree essential oil

Instructions:

1. **Mix Ingredients:** In a spray bottle, combine 1 tablespoon of castor oil, 2 tablespoons of aloe vera juice, and 1 cup of distilled water.
2. **Add Essential Oil:** Add 10 drops of tea tree essential oil to the spray bottle.
3. **Shake Well:** Shake the bottle well to mix the ingredients thoroughly.

How to Use:

1. **Apply to Damp Hair:** After washing your hair, spray the leave-in conditioner evenly onto your damp hair.
2. **Distribute Evenly:** Use a wide-tooth comb to distribute the spray throughout your hair, focusing on the ends and any tangled areas.
3. **Style as Usual:** Let your hair air dry or style as usual.

Benefits:

-   **Hydrates:** Aloe vera juice and castor oil provide hydration to keep hair soft and manageable.
-   **Detangles:** The leave-in formula helps detangle hair, reducing breakage and making it easier to comb.

4. Castor Oil Shine Spray

Purpose: To add shine and smoothness to hair.

Ingredients:

-   1 tablespoon of castor oil
-   1 tablespoon of jojoba oil
-   1/2 cup of distilled water
-   5 drops of ylang-ylang essential oil

Instructions:

1. **Mix Ingredients:** In a spray bottle, combine 1 tablespoon of castor oil, 1 tablespoon of jojoba oil, and 1/2 cup of distilled water.
2. **Add Essential Oil:** Add 5 drops of ylang-ylang essential oil to the spray bottle.
3. **Shake Well:** Shake the bottle well to mix the ingredients thoroughly.

How to Use:

1. **Apply to Dry Hair:** Spray the shine spray lightly onto dry hair, focusing on the mid-lengths and ends.
2. **Distribute Evenly:** Use your fingers to distribute the spray and smooth down any flyaways.
3. **Style as Usual:** Style your hair as desired.

Benefits:

- **Adds Shine:** Jojoba oil and ylang-ylang essential oil add a beautiful shine to the hair.
- **Smooths Hair:** Helps smooth the hair cuticle, reducing frizz and flyaways.

5. Castor Oil Scalp Treatment Spray

Purpose: To soothe the scalp and promote a healthy environment for hair growth.

Ingredients:

- 2 tablespoons of castor oil
- 1 tablespoon of witch hazel
- 1/2 cup of distilled water
- 10 drops of peppermint essential oil

Instructions:

1. **Mix Ingredients:** In a spray bottle, combine 2 tablespoons of castor oil, 1 tablespoon of witch hazel, and 1/2 cup of distilled water.
2. **Add Essential Oil:** Add 10 drops of peppermint essential oil to the spray bottle.
3. **Shake Well:** Shake the bottle well to mix the ingredients thoroughly.

How to Use:

1. **Apply to Scalp:** Spray the scalp treatment directly onto your scalp, parting your hair in sections to ensure even coverage.
2. **Massage:** Gently massage the spray into your scalp for 5-10 minutes.
3. **Leave On:** Leave the treatment on for at least 30 minutes before washing your hair. For best results, leave it on overnight.
4. **Frequency:** Use the scalp treatment 1-2 times a week.

Benefits:

- **Soothes Scalp:** Witch hazel and peppermint essential oil soothe and cool the scalp, reducing inflammation and irritation.
- **Promotes Growth:** Castor oil promotes a healthy scalp environment, supporting hair growth.

Application methods

Proper application methods are crucial to maximizing the benefits of castor oil serums and sprays. These methods ensure even distribution, optimal absorption, and effective results. Here's an in-depth guide on how to apply each of the castor oil serums and sprays effectively.

1. Castor Oil Hair Growth Serum

Purpose: To promote hair growth and strengthen hair.

Application Steps:

1. **Prepare Your Hair:** Start with clean, dry hair to ensure the serum penetrates effectively.
2. **Section Your Hair:** Use a comb to part your hair into small sections. This helps ensure the serum reaches the scalp evenly.
3. **Apply the Serum:** Use the dropper to apply a few drops of the serum directly onto your scalp, focusing on one section at a time.
4. **Massage the Scalp:** Gently massage the serum into your scalp using circular motions. Spend about 5-10 minutes massaging to stimulate blood circulation and enhance absorption.
5. **Leave On:** For best results, leave the serum on overnight or for at least 1-2 hours before washing your hair.
6. **Frequency:** Use the serum 2-3 times a week for optimal hair growth benefits.

2. Castor Oil Anti-Frizz Serum

Purpose: To tame frizz and add shine.

Application Steps:

1. **Prepare Your Hair:** After washing your hair, towel-dry it until it's damp but not dripping wet.
2. **Apply the Serum:** Pump a small amount of the serum into your palms. Rub your hands together to distribute the serum evenly.
3. **Distribute Evenly:** Apply the serum to your hair, starting from the mid-lengths to the ends. Avoid applying too much to the roots to prevent greasiness.
4. **Focus on Frizzy Areas:** Pay extra attention to any frizzy or flyaway-prone areas.
5. **Style as Usual:** Let your hair air dry or style it as usual. The serum will help keep your hair smooth and shiny.

3. Castor Oil Leave-In Conditioning Spray

Purpose: To hydrate and detangle hair.

Application Steps:

1. **Prepare Your Hair:** After washing your hair, towel-dry it until it's damp.
2. **Shake Well:** Before each use, shake the spray bottle well to ensure the ingredients are thoroughly mixed.
3. **Spray Evenly:** Hold the spray bottle about 6-8 inches away from your hair and spray the leave-in conditioner evenly. Focus on the mid-lengths to the ends.
4. **Detangle:** Use a wide-tooth comb to gently detangle your hair, ensuring the spray is evenly distributed.

5. **Style as Usual:** Let your hair air dry or style it as desired. The leave-in conditioner will keep your hair hydrated and manageable.

4. Castor Oil Shine Spray

Purpose: To add shine and smoothness to hair.

Application Steps:

1. **Prepare Your Hair:** Use the shine spray on dry hair for best results.
2. **Shake Well:** Shake the spray bottle well before each use to mix the ingredients.
3. **Spray Lightly:** Hold the spray bottle about 6-8 inches away from your hair and spray lightly. Focus on the mid-lengths to the ends for a natural shine.
4. **Smooth Down:** Use your fingers to smooth down any flyaways and distribute the spray evenly.
5. **Style as Usual:** Style your hair as desired. The shine spray will add a healthy, glossy finish to your hair.

5. Castor Oil Scalp Treatment Spray

Purpose: To soothe the scalp and promote a healthy environment for hair growth.

Application Steps:

1. **Prepare Your Hair:** Apply the scalp treatment spray to clean, dry hair for the best absorption.
2. **Section Your Hair:** Use a comb to part your hair into small sections to ensure the spray reaches the scalp evenly.
3. **Spray Directly:** Hold the spray bottle close to your scalp and spray directly onto the scalp. Focus on one section at a time for thorough coverage.
4. **Massage the Scalp:** Gently massage the spray into your scalp using circular motions for 5-10 minutes. This enhances blood flow and helps the treatment absorb better.
5. **Leave On:** Leave the treatment on for at least 30 minutes, or overnight for deeper treatment. Wash your hair afterward if leaving it on overnight.
6. **Frequency:** Use the scalp treatment 1-2 times a week to maintain a healthy scalp and promote hair growth.

General Tips for All Applications:

1. Clean Hair: Always start with clean hair to ensure that the oils and treatments penetrate effectively without the interference of dirt or product buildup. **2. Even Distribution:** Ensure even distribution of the product to maximize its effectiveness. Use combs, fingers, or sectioning techniques to cover all areas. **3. Gentle Handling:** Be gentle when massaging or combing your hair to avoid breakage and hair loss. **4. Regular Use:** Consistency is key. Regular use of these serums and sprays will provide the best results. **5. Storage:** Store your DIY products in a cool, dark place to maintain their potency and extend their shelf life.

Part IV

Enhancing the Effects of Castor Oil

Combining Castor Oil with Other Ingredients

Essential Oils

Benefits and combinations

Combining castor oil with essential oils can enhance its effectiveness and add additional benefits for hair care. Essential oils are known for their unique properties, such as promoting hair growth, soothing the scalp, and adding fragrance. Here's an in-depth look at the benefits of using essential oils with castor oil and some effective combinations.

1. Rosemary Essential Oil

Benefits:

- **Stimulates Hair Growth:** Rosemary oil is known to improve circulation to the scalp, promoting hair growth and preventing hair loss.
- **Strengthens Hair:** It strengthens hair follicles, helping to reduce breakage and thinning.
- **Reduces Dandruff:** Its antifungal properties help combat dandruff and maintain scalp health.

Combination with Castor Oil:

- **Hair Growth Serum:** Mix 2 tablespoons of castor oil with 10 drops of rosemary essential oil. Apply to the scalp and massage for 5-10 minutes. Leave on for at least an hour before washing.
- **Overnight Treatment:** Combine 2 tablespoons of castor oil with 10 drops of rosemary oil and leave the mixture on overnight for a deep conditioning treatment.

2. Lavender Essential Oil

Benefits:

- **Promotes Hair Growth:** Lavender oil can stimulate hair growth and increase the number of hair follicles.
- **Calms and Soothes:** It has calming properties that can reduce stress, which is often linked to hair loss.
- **Antimicrobial:** Lavender oil has antimicrobial properties that can prevent bacteria and fungi from growing on the scalp.

Combination with Castor Oil:

- **Anti-Frizz Serum:** Mix 1 tablespoon of castor oil with 1 tablespoon of argan oil and 5 drops of lavender essential oil. Apply to damp hair, focusing on frizzy areas.
- **Scalp Treatment:** Combine 2 tablespoons of castor oil with 10 drops of lavender oil. Massage into the scalp and leave on for an hour before washing.

3. Peppermint Essential Oil

Benefits:

- **Stimulates Circulation:** Peppermint oil increases blood flow to the scalp, which can promote hair growth.
- **Cools and Soothes:** Its cooling effect can soothe itching and inflammation.
- **Antibacterial:** Peppermint oil has antibacterial properties that help maintain a healthy scalp.

Combination with Castor Oil:

- **Scalp Treatment Spray:** Mix 2 tablespoons of castor oil with 1 tablespoon of witch hazel, 1/2 cup of distilled water, and 10 drops of peppermint essential oil. Spray directly onto the scalp and massage.
- **Hair Growth Serum:** Combine 2 tablespoons of castor oil with 10 drops of peppermint oil. Apply to the scalp and leave on overnight.

4. Tea Tree Essential Oil

Benefits:

- **Fights Dandruff:** Tea tree oil is effective against dandruff due to its antifungal and antibacterial properties.
- **Reduces Scalp Inflammation:** It soothes inflammation and can help with conditions like seborrheic dermatitis.
- **Promotes Hair Growth:** By maintaining a healthy scalp, tea tree oil supports healthy hair growth.

Combination with Castor Oil:

- **Leave-In Conditioning Spray:** Mix 1 tablespoon of castor oil, 2 tablespoons of aloe vera juice, 1 cup of distilled water, and 10 drops of tea tree essential oil. Spray onto damp hair and comb through.
- **Dandruff Treatment:** Combine 2 tablespoons of castor oil with 10 drops of tea tree oil. Massage into the scalp and leave on for an hour before washing.

5. Ylang-Ylang Essential Oil

Benefits:

- **Balances Oil Production:** Ylang-ylang oil helps balance sebum production, making it beneficial for both dry and oily scalps.
- **Improves Hair Texture:** It conditions the hair, making it smoother and more manageable.
- **Reduces Hair Breakage:** Strengthens hair and reduces breakage.

Combination with Castor Oil:

- **Shine Spray:** Mix 1 tablespoon of castor oil, 1 tablespoon of jojoba oil, 1/2 cup of distilled water, and 5 drops of ylang-ylang essential oil. Spray onto dry hair for added shine.
- **Deep Conditioning Mask:** Combine 2 tablespoons of castor oil with 10 drops of ylang-ylang oil. Apply to hair and scalp, cover with a shower cap, and leave on for an hour before rinsing.

6. Cedarwood Essential Oil

Benefits:

- **Stimulates Hair Growth:** Cedarwood oil stimulates hair follicles by increasing circulation to the scalp.
- **Antiseptic Properties:** It has antiseptic properties that help maintain scalp health.
- **Balances Oil Production:** Cedarwood oil helps balance the oil-producing glands in the scalp.

Combination with Castor Oil:

- **Hair Growth Serum:** Mix 2 tablespoons of castor oil with 10 drops of cedarwood essential oil. Massage into the scalp and leave on overnight.
- **Scalp Health Treatment:** Combine 2 tablespoons of castor oil with 10 drops of cedarwood oil. Apply to the scalp and leave on for an hour before washing.

Application techniques

Proper application techniques are crucial for maximizing the benefits of castor oil combined with essential oils. These methods ensure that the oils are absorbed effectively, providing the desired benefits for hair and scalp health. Here's a comprehensive guide on how to apply these mixtures for optimal results.

1. Hair Growth Serum with Rosemary Essential Oil

Purpose: To promote hair growth and strengthen hair.

Application Steps:

1. **Prepare the Serum:** Mix 2 tablespoons of castor oil with 10 drops of rosemary essential oil in a small bottle with a dropper.
2. **Section Your Hair:** Use a comb to part your hair into small sections. This helps ensure the serum reaches the scalp evenly.
3. **Apply the Serum:** Use the dropper to apply a few drops of the serum directly onto your scalp, focusing on one section at a time.

4. **Massage the Scalp:** Gently massage the serum into your scalp using circular motions for 5-10 minutes. This stimulates blood circulation and enhances absorption.
5. **Leave On:** For best results, leave the serum on overnight or for at least 1-2 hours before washing your hair.
6. **Frequency:** Use the serum 2-3 times a week for optimal hair growth benefits.

2. Anti-Frizz Serum with Lavender Essential Oil

Purpose: To tame frizz and add shine.

Application Steps:

1. **Prepare the Serum:** Mix 1 tablespoon of castor oil with 1 tablespoon of argan oil and 5 drops of lavender essential oil in a small bottle with a pump.
2. **Apply to Damp Hair:** After washing your hair, towel-dry it until it's damp but not dripping wet.
3. **Distribute Evenly:** Pump a small amount of the serum into your palms. Rub your hands together to distribute the serum evenly, then apply it to your hair, starting from the mid-lengths to the ends. Avoid applying too much to the roots to prevent greasiness.
4. **Style as Usual:** Let your hair air dry or style it as usual. The serum will help keep your hair smooth and shiny.

3. Leave-In Conditioning Spray with Tea Tree Essential Oil

Purpose: To hydrate and detangle hair.

Application Steps:

1. **Prepare the Spray:** In a spray bottle, mix 1 tablespoon of castor oil, 2 tablespoons of aloe vera juice, 1 cup of distilled water, and 10 drops of tea tree essential oil.
2. **Shake Well:** Shake the spray bottle well before each use to ensure the ingredients are thoroughly mixed.
3. **Spray Evenly:** Hold the spray bottle about 6-8 inches away from your hair and spray the leave-in conditioner evenly onto your damp hair.
4. **Detangle:** Use a wide-tooth comb to gently detangle your hair, ensuring the spray is evenly distributed.
5. **Style as Usual:** Let your hair air dry or style it as desired. The leave-in conditioner will keep your hair hydrated and manageable.

4. Shine Spray with Ylang-Ylang Essential Oil

Purpose: To add shine and smoothness to hair.

Application Steps:

1. **Prepare the Spray:** Mix 1 tablespoon of castor oil, 1 tablespoon of jojoba oil, 1/2 cup of distilled water, and 5 drops of ylang-ylang essential oil in a spray bottle.

2. **Shake Well:** Shake the spray bottle well before each use to mix the ingredients.
3. **Spray Lightly:** Hold the spray bottle about 6-8 inches away from your hair and spray lightly, focusing on the mid-lengths to the ends for a natural shine.
4. **Smooth Down:** Use your fingers to smooth down any flyaways and distribute the spray evenly.
5. **Style as Usual:** Style your hair as desired. The shine spray will add a healthy, glossy finish to your hair.

5. Scalp Treatment Spray with Peppermint Essential Oil

Purpose: To soothe the scalp and promote a healthy environment for hair growth.

Application Steps:

1. **Prepare the Spray:** Mix 2 tablespoons of castor oil, 1 tablespoon of witch hazel, 1/2 cup of distilled water, and 10 drops of peppermint essential oil in a spray bottle.
2. **Shake Well:** Shake the spray bottle well before each use to ensure the ingredients are thoroughly mixed.
3. **Apply to Scalp:** Hold the spray bottle close to your scalp and spray directly onto the scalp, parting your hair in sections to ensure even coverage.
4. **Massage the Scalp:** Gently massage the spray into your scalp using circular motions for 5-10 minutes. This enhances blood flow and helps the treatment absorb better.
5. **Leave On:** Leave the treatment on for at least 30 minutes, or overnight for deeper treatment. Wash your hair afterward if leaving it on overnight.
6. **Frequency:** Use the scalp treatment 1-2 times a week to maintain a healthy scalp and promote hair growth.

General Tips for All Applications:

1. Clean Hair: Always start with clean hair to ensure that the oils and treatments penetrate effectively without the interference of dirt or product buildup. **2. Even Distribution:** Ensure even distribution of the product to maximize its effectiveness. Use combs, fingers, or sectioning techniques to cover all areas. **3. Gentle Handling:** Be gentle when massaging or combing your hair to avoid breakage and hair loss. **4. Regular Use:** Consistency is key. Regular use of these serums and sprays will provide the best results. **5. Storage:** Store your DIY products in a cool, dark place to maintain their potency and extend their shelf life.

Carrier Oils

Best carrier oils to use

Carrier oils are base oils used to dilute essential oils and castor oil, making them easier to apply and enhancing their benefits. Each carrier oil offers unique properties that complement castor oil, providing additional nourishment, hydration, and protection for your hair and scalp. Here's a detailed guide to the best carrier oils to use with castor oil and their benefits.

1. Coconut Oil

Benefits:

- **Deep Moisturization:** Coconut oil penetrates the hair shaft deeply, providing intense hydration and preventing dryness.
- **Strengthens Hair:** Rich in fatty acids, coconut oil strengthens hair and reduces protein loss.
- **Anti-Fungal Properties:** Helps combat dandruff and scalp infections due to its anti-fungal properties.

How to Use:

- **Mixing Ratio:** Combine equal parts of castor oil and coconut oil. Warm the mixture slightly before application for better absorption.
- **Application:** Apply to the scalp and hair, focusing on the ends. Leave on for at least 30 minutes or overnight for deep conditioning.

2. Jojoba Oil

Benefits:

- **Balancing Oil Production:** Jojoba oil closely resembles the scalp's natural sebum, helping to balance oil production.
- **Moisturizes Scalp:** Keeps the scalp hydrated without leaving a greasy residue.
- **Nourishes Hair:** Rich in vitamins E and B, jojoba oil nourishes hair and promotes healthy growth.

How to Use:

- **Mixing Ratio:** Mix 2 tablespoons of castor oil with 1 tablespoon of jojoba oil.
- **Application:** Apply to the scalp and hair, massaging gently. Leave on for at least an hour before washing.

3. Argan Oil

Benefits:

- **Hydrates and Softens:** Argan oil is rich in essential fatty acids and vitamin E, providing deep hydration and making hair softer.
- **Adds Shine:** Adds a natural shine to the hair, making it look healthier and more vibrant.
- **Protects from Damage:** Protects hair from environmental damage and heat styling.

How to Use:

- **Mixing Ratio:** Combine 2 tablespoons of castor oil with 1 tablespoon of argan oil.
- **Application:** Apply to damp or dry hair, focusing on the mid-lengths and ends. Leave on for 30 minutes before washing.

4. Olive Oil

Benefits:

- **Strengthens Hair:** Olive oil is rich in antioxidants and vitamin E, which strengthen hair and promote growth.
- **Moisturizes:** Provides deep moisture, making hair more manageable and reducing frizz.
- **Improves Scalp Health:** Helps maintain a healthy scalp by reducing dandruff and soothing irritation.

How to Use:

- **Mixing Ratio:** Mix equal parts of castor oil and olive oil.
- **Application:** Apply to the scalp and hair, massaging gently. Leave on for at least an hour or overnight before washing.

5. Almond Oil

Benefits:

- **Nourishes Hair:** Almond oil is rich in vitamins A, B, and E, which nourish and strengthen hair.
- **Reduces Hair Loss:** Helps reduce hair loss by making hair stronger and less prone to breakage.
- **Improves Shine:** Adds a natural shine and smoothness to the hair.

How to Use:

- **Mixing Ratio:** Combine 2 tablespoons of castor oil with 1 tablespoon of almond oil.
- **Application:** Apply to the scalp and hair, focusing on the roots and ends. Leave on for 30 minutes before washing.

6. Grapeseed Oil

Benefits:

- **Lightweight Moisturization:** Grapeseed oil is lightweight and easily absorbed, providing moisture without weighing hair down.
- **Strengthens Hair:** Contains antioxidants and essential fatty acids that strengthen hair and promote growth.
- **Reduces Dandruff:** Helps reduce dandruff and maintains a healthy scalp.

How to Use:

- **Mixing Ratio:** Mix 2 tablespoons of castor oil with 1 tablespoon of grapeseed oil.
- **Application:** Apply to the scalp and hair, massaging gently. Leave on for at least 30 minutes before washing.

7. Avocado Oil

Benefits:

- **Deep Conditioning:** Avocado oil penetrates deeply into the hair shaft, providing intense conditioning and moisture.
- **Rich in Nutrients:** Contains vitamins A, D, E, and B6, as well as folic acid and amino acids, which nourish hair.
- **Reduces Damage:** Helps repair and protect hair from damage caused by environmental factors and heat styling.

How to Use:

- **Mixing Ratio:** Combine equal parts of castor oil and avocado oil.
- **Application:** Apply to the scalp and hair, focusing on the ends. Leave on for 30 minutes or overnight for deep conditioning.

General Tips for Using Carrier Oils with Castor Oil:

1. Warm the Mixture: Warming the oil mixture slightly before application can enhance absorption and make it easier to apply. **2. Consistent Use:** Regular use of these oil blends can provide long-term benefits for hair and scalp health. **3. Scalp Massage:** Always massage the oil into your scalp to stimulate blood flow and enhance absorption. **4. Leave-On Time:** For deep conditioning, leave the oil mixture on for at least 30 minutes or overnight. **5. Rinse Thoroughly:** Ensure thorough rinsing and shampooing to remove all traces of oil.

Mixing ratios and benefits

Combining castor oil with different carrier oils can enhance the effectiveness of your hair care treatments. Each carrier oil brings its unique properties, making it important to understand the optimal mixing ratios and the specific benefits they offer. Here's a detailed guide on how to mix castor oil with various carrier oils and the benefits of each combination.

1. Castor Oil and Coconut Oil

Mixing Ratio:

- **Equal Parts:** Mix equal parts of castor oil and coconut oil.

Benefits:

- **Deep Moisturization:** Coconut oil penetrates deeply into the hair shaft, providing intense hydration and preventing dryness.
- **Strengthens Hair:** The combination helps reduce protein loss, strengthening the hair and reducing breakage.

- **Anti-Fungal Properties:** Coconut oil's anti-fungal properties help combat dandruff and scalp infections, maintaining a healthy scalp environment.

2. Castor Oil and Jojoba Oil

Mixing Ratio:

- **2:1 Ratio:** Mix 2 tablespoons of castor oil with 1 tablespoon of jojoba oil.

Benefits:

- **Balances Oil Production:** Jojoba oil closely resembles the scalp's natural sebum, helping to balance oil production and prevent scalp issues.
- **Moisturizes Scalp:** Keeps the scalp hydrated without leaving a greasy residue, promoting a healthy scalp environment.
- **Nourishes Hair:** Rich in vitamins E and B, jojoba oil nourishes hair, promoting healthy growth and reducing hair loss.

3. Castor Oil and Argan Oil

Mixing Ratio:

- **2:1 Ratio:** Mix 2 tablespoons of castor oil with 1 tablespoon of argan oil.

Benefits:

- **Hydrates and Softens:** Argan oil provides deep hydration, making hair softer and more manageable.
- **Adds Shine:** The combination adds a natural shine to the hair, enhancing its overall appearance.
- **Protects from Damage:** Argan oil helps protect hair from environmental damage and heat styling, keeping it healthy and resilient.

4. Castor Oil and Olive Oil

Mixing Ratio:

- **Equal Parts:** Mix equal parts of castor oil and olive oil.

Benefits:

- **Strengthens Hair:** Olive oil is rich in antioxidants and vitamin E, which strengthen hair and promote growth.
- **Moisturizes:** Provides deep moisture, reducing frizz and making hair more manageable.
- **Improves Scalp Health:** Olive oil helps maintain a healthy scalp by reducing dandruff and soothing irritation.

5. Castor Oil and Almond Oil

Mixing Ratio:

- **2:1 Ratio:** Mix 2 tablespoons of castor oil with 1 tablespoon of almond oil.

Benefits:

- **Nourishes Hair:** Almond oil is rich in vitamins A, B, and E, which nourish and strengthen hair, reducing breakage.
- **Reduces Hair Loss:** Helps reduce hair loss by making hair stronger and less prone to damage.
- **Improves Shine:** Adds a natural shine and smoothness to the hair, enhancing its overall look and feel.

6. Castor Oil and Grapeseed Oil

Mixing Ratio:

- **2:1 Ratio:** Mix 2 tablespoons of castor oil with 1 tablespoon of grapeseed oil.

Benefits:

- **Lightweight Moisturization:** Grapeseed oil is lightweight and easily absorbed, providing moisture without weighing hair down.
- **Strengthens Hair:** Contains antioxidants and essential fatty acids that strengthen hair and promote growth.
- **Reduces Dandruff:** Helps reduce dandruff and maintains a healthy scalp environment.

7. Castor Oil and Avocado Oil

Mixing Ratio:

- **Equal Parts:** Mix equal parts of castor oil and avocado oil.

Benefits:

- **Deep Conditioning:** Avocado oil penetrates deeply into the hair shaft, providing intense conditioning and moisture.
- **Rich in Nutrients:** Contains vitamins A, D, E, and B6, as well as folic acid and amino acids, which nourish hair and promote health.
- **Reduces Damage:** Helps repair and protect hair from damage caused by environmental factors and heat styling.

General Tips for Mixing and Using Castor Oil with Carrier Oils:

1. Warm the Mixture: Slightly warming the oil mixture before application can enhance absorption and make it easier to apply. **2. Consistent Use:** Regular use of these oil blends can provide long-term benefits for hair and scalp health. **3. Scalp Massage:** Always massage the oil into your scalp to stimulate blood flow and enhance absorption. **4. Leave-On Time:** For deep conditioning, leave the oil mixture on for at least 30 minutes or overnight. **5. Rinse Thoroughly:** Ensure thorough rinsing and shampooing to remove all traces of oil.

Herbal Infusions

Herbs that complement castor oil

Herbal infusions can significantly enhance the benefits of castor oil for hair and scalp care. Various herbs offer unique properties that complement castor oil, providing additional nourishment, stimulating hair growth, and improving scalp health. Here's a detailed guide on the best herbs to use with castor oil and their benefits.

1. Rosemary

Benefits:

- **Stimulates Hair Growth:** Rosemary is known for its ability to improve blood circulation to the scalp, which can stimulate hair growth and prevent hair loss.
- **Strengthens Hair:** Helps strengthen hair follicles, reducing hair breakage and thinning.
- **Antioxidant Properties:** Rich in antioxidants, rosemary helps fight free radicals that can damage hair cells.

How to Use:

- **Infusion Method:** Boil a handful of fresh or dried rosemary leaves in water. Let it cool, strain, and mix the rosemary water with castor oil in equal parts.
- **Application:** Apply the mixture to your scalp and hair, massage gently, and leave on for 30 minutes to an hour before washing.

2. Lavender

Benefits:

- **Promotes Hair Growth:** Lavender can stimulate hair growth and increase the number of hair follicles.
- **Calms and Soothes:** Its calming properties can reduce stress, which is often linked to hair loss.
- **Antimicrobial:** Lavender's antimicrobial properties help prevent bacteria and fungi from growing on the scalp.

How to Use:

- **Infusion Method:** Steep lavender flowers in boiling water for 10-15 minutes. Let it cool, strain, and mix the lavender water with castor oil.

- **Application:** Apply the mixture to your scalp and hair, massage, and leave on for at least 30 minutes before rinsing.

3. Peppermint

Benefits:

- **Stimulates Circulation:** Peppermint increases blood flow to the scalp, promoting hair growth.
- **Cools and Soothes:** Provides a cooling effect that soothes itching and inflammation.
- **Antibacterial:** Helps maintain a healthy scalp with its antibacterial properties.

How to Use:

- **Infusion Method:** Boil a handful of peppermint leaves in water. Let it cool, strain, and mix the peppermint water with castor oil.
- **Application:** Apply to the scalp and hair, massage, and leave on for 30 minutes to an hour before washing.

4. Chamomile

Benefits:

- **Soothes Scalp:** Chamomile is known for its soothing properties, reducing scalp irritation and inflammation.
- **Adds Shine:** Helps add shine and softness to the hair.
- **Promotes Hair Growth:** Encourages healthy hair growth by maintaining a healthy scalp environment.

How to Use:

- **Infusion Method:** Steep chamomile flowers in boiling water for 10-15 minutes. Let it cool, strain, and mix the chamomile water with castor oil.
- **Application:** Apply the mixture to your scalp and hair, massage, and leave on for at least 30 minutes before rinsing.

5. Nettle

Benefits:

- **Strengthens Hair:** Nettle is rich in vitamins and minerals that strengthen hair and promote growth.
- **Reduces Hair Loss:** Helps reduce hair loss by stimulating the scalp and improving blood circulation.
- **Anti-Inflammatory:** Its anti-inflammatory properties help soothe the scalp.

How to Use:

- **Infusion Method:** Boil nettle leaves in water for 10-15 minutes. Let it cool, strain, and mix the nettle water with castor oil.
- **Application:** Apply to the scalp and hair, massage, and leave on for at least 30 minutes before rinsing.

6. Sage

Benefits:

- **Promotes Hair Growth:** Sage helps stimulate hair growth by improving circulation to the scalp.
- **Cleanses Scalp:** Has cleansing properties that help remove buildup and maintain a healthy scalp.
- **Adds Shine:** Leaves hair looking shiny and healthy.

How to Use:

- **Infusion Method:** Steep sage leaves in boiling water for 10-15 minutes. Let it cool, strain, and mix the sage water with castor oil.
- **Application:** Apply the mixture to your scalp and hair, massage, and leave on for at least 30 minutes before rinsing.

7. Horsetail

Benefits:

- **Strengthens Hair:** Horsetail is high in silica, which strengthens hair and improves its texture.
- **Promotes Hair Growth:** Encourages hair growth by stimulating the scalp.
- **Prevents Hair Loss:** Helps prevent hair loss by maintaining a healthy scalp environment.

How to Use:

- **Infusion Method:** Boil horsetail in water for 10-15 minutes. Let it cool, strain, and mix the horsetail water with castor oil.
- **Application:** Apply to the scalp and hair, massage, and leave on for at least 30 minutes before rinsing.

General Tips for Using Herbal Infusions with Castor Oil:

1. Fresh or Dried Herbs: Both fresh and dried herbs can be used to make infusions. Fresh herbs are often more potent, but dried herbs can be more convenient. **2. Proper Straining:** Ensure the herbal infusion is well-strained to avoid bits of herbs getting stuck in your hair. **3. Warm the Mixture:** Slightly warming the mixture before application can enhance absorption. **4. Consistent Use:** Regular use of these herbal infusions can provide long-term benefits for hair and scalp health. **5. Scalp Massage:** Always massage the mixture into your scalp to stimulate blood flow and enhance absorption.

Preparation methods

To maximize the benefits of combining castor oil with herbal infusions, it's important to understand the proper preparation methods. These methods ensure that the nutrients from the herbs are effectively extracted and combined with castor oil to enhance their effectiveness. Here's a detailed guide on how to prepare and use herbal infusions with castor oil.

1. Basic Herbal Infusion Preparation

Ingredients:

- Fresh or dried herbs (rosemary, lavender, peppermint, chamomile, nettle, sage, horsetail)
- Water
- Castor oil

Equipment:

- Saucepan or kettle
- Strainer or cheesecloth
- Mixing bowl
- Storage container (bottle or jar)

Steps:

1. **Boil the Water:** Bring a pot of water to a boil. Use about 2 cups of water for every handful of fresh herbs or 2 tablespoons of dried herbs.
2. **Add the Herbs:** Once the water is boiling, remove it from the heat and add the herbs. Stir to ensure they are fully submerged.
3. **Steep the Herbs:** Cover the pot and let the herbs steep for 15-30 minutes. This allows the beneficial compounds to be extracted into the water.
4. **Strain the Infusion:** After steeping, strain the liquid through a fine strainer or cheesecloth into a mixing bowl to remove the herbs.
5. **Cool the Infusion:** Allow the herbal infusion to cool to room temperature.
6. **Mix with Castor Oil:** Combine the herbal infusion with castor oil in equal parts. For example, if you have 1 cup of herbal infusion, mix it with 1 cup of castor oil.
7. **Store the Mixture:** Pour the mixture into a clean bottle or jar for storage. Shake well before each use.

2. Rosemary and Castor Oil Infusion

Purpose: To stimulate hair growth and strengthen hair.

Ingredients:

- Fresh or dried rosemary
- Water
- Castor oil

Steps:

1. **Prepare the Infusion:** Boil 2 cups of water and add a handful of fresh rosemary or 2 tablespoons of dried rosemary. Remove from heat and steep for 20 minutes.
2. **Strain and Cool:** Strain the infusion and let it cool to room temperature.
3. **Mix with Castor Oil:** Combine 1 cup of rosemary infusion with 1 cup of castor oil. Mix well.
4. **Application:** Apply to the scalp and hair, massage gently, and leave on for 30 minutes to an hour before washing.

3. Lavender and Castor Oil Infusion

Purpose: To promote hair growth and calm the scalp.

Ingredients:

- Fresh or dried lavender
- Water
- Castor oil

Steps:

1. **Prepare the Infusion:** Boil 2 cups of water and add a handful of fresh lavender or 2 tablespoons of dried lavender. Remove from heat and steep for 15 minutes.
2. **Strain and Cool:** Strain the infusion and let it cool to room temperature.
3. **Mix with Castor Oil:** Combine 1 cup of lavender infusion with 1 cup of castor oil. Mix well.
4. **Application:** Apply to the scalp and hair, massage gently, and leave on for at least 30 minutes before rinsing.

4. Peppermint and Castor Oil Infusion

Purpose: To stimulate circulation and soothe the scalp.

Ingredients:

- Fresh or dried peppermint
- Water
- Castor oil

Steps:

1. **Prepare the Infusion:** Boil 2 cups of water and add a handful of fresh peppermint or 2 tablespoons of dried peppermint. Remove from heat and steep for 20 minutes.
2. **Strain and Cool:** Strain the infusion and let it cool to room temperature.
3. **Mix with Castor Oil:** Combine 1 cup of peppermint infusion with 1 cup of castor oil. Mix well.

4. **Application:** Apply to the scalp and hair, massage gently, and leave on for 30 minutes to an hour before washing.

5. Chamomile and Castor Oil Infusion

Purpose: To soothe the scalp and add shine to hair.

Ingredients:

- Fresh or dried chamomile
- Water
- Castor oil

Steps:

1. **Prepare the Infusion:** Boil 2 cups of water and add a handful of fresh chamomile or 2 tablespoons of dried chamomile. Remove from heat and steep for 15 minutes.
2. **Strain and Cool:** Strain the infusion and let it cool to room temperature.
3. **Mix with Castor Oil:** Combine 1 cup of chamomile infusion with 1 cup of castor oil. Mix well.
4. **Application:** Apply to the scalp and hair, massage gently, and leave on for at least 30 minutes before rinsing.

6. Nettle and Castor Oil Infusion

Purpose: To strengthen hair and reduce hair loss.

Ingredients:

- Fresh or dried nettle
- Water
- Castor oil

Steps:

1. **Prepare the Infusion:** Boil 2 cups of water and add a handful of fresh nettle or 2 tablespoons of dried nettle. Remove from heat and steep for 20 minutes.
2. **Strain and Cool:** Strain the infusion and let it cool to room temperature.
3. **Mix with Castor Oil:** Combine 1 cup of nettle infusion with 1 cup of castor oil. Mix well.
4. **Application:** Apply to the scalp and hair, massage gently, and leave on for at least 30 minutes before rinsing.

7. Sage and Castor Oil Infusion

Purpose: To promote hair growth and cleanse the scalp.

Ingredients:

- Fresh or dried sage

- Water
- Castor oil

Steps:

1. **Prepare the Infusion:** Boil 2 cups of water and add a handful of fresh sage or 2 tablespoons of dried sage. Remove from heat and steep for 15 minutes.
2. **Strain and Cool:** Strain the infusion and let it cool to room temperature.
3. **Mix with Castor Oil:** Combine 1 cup of sage infusion with 1 cup of castor oil. Mix well.
4. **Application:** Apply to the scalp and hair, massage gently, and leave on for at least 30 minutes before rinsing.

8. Horsetail and Castor Oil Infusion

Purpose: To strengthen hair and promote growth.

Ingredients:

- Fresh or dried horsetail
- Water
- Castor oil

Steps:

1. **Prepare the Infusion:** Boil 2 cups of water and add a handful of fresh horsetail or 2 tablespoons of dried horsetail. Remove from heat and steep for 20 minutes.
2. **Strain and Cool:** Strain the infusion and let it cool to room temperature.
3. **Mix with Castor Oil:** Combine 1 cup of horsetail infusion with 1 cup of castor oil. Mix well.
4. **Application:** Apply to the scalp and hair, massage gently, and leave on for at least 30 minutes before rinsing.

General Tips for Preparing Herbal Infusions with Castor Oil:

1. Fresh or Dried Herbs: Both fresh and dried herbs can be used for infusions. Fresh herbs often provide more potent infusions, while dried herbs are more convenient and have a longer shelf life. **2. Proper Straining:** Ensure the herbal infusion is well-strained to avoid bits of herbs getting stuck in your hair. **3. Warm the Mixture:** Slightly warming the mixture before application can enhance absorption. **4. Consistent Use:** Regular use of these herbal infusions can provide long-term benefits for hair and scalp health. **5. Scalp Massage:** Always massage the mixture into your scalp to stimulate blood flow and enhance absorption.

Healthy Lifestyle Practices for Hair Growth

Diet and Nutrition

Foods that promote hair health

A healthy diet rich in essential nutrients is crucial for promoting hair growth and maintaining overall hair health. Certain foods contain vitamins, minerals, and other compounds that are particularly beneficial for hair. Here's a detailed guide on the best foods to include in your diet to support healthy hair growth.

1. Salmon

Nutrient Benefits:

- **Omega-3 Fatty Acids:** Salmon is rich in omega-3 fatty acids, which nourish the hair follicles and promote healthy hair growth.
- **Protein:** Provides high-quality protein that strengthens hair and prevents breakage.
- **Vitamin D:** Helps create new hair follicles, which can improve hair thickness.

How to Include:

- **Grilled or Baked:** Incorporate salmon into your diet by grilling or baking it for a nutritious meal.
- **Salmon Salad:** Add cooked salmon to salads for a protein-rich addition.
- **Smoked Salmon:** Enjoy smoked salmon on whole-grain toast for a healthy breakfast or snack.

2. Eggs

Nutrient Benefits:

- **Biotin:** Eggs are an excellent source of biotin, a B vitamin that promotes hair growth and helps prevent hair loss.
- **Protein:** Rich in high-quality protein, which is essential for hair structure.
- **Zinc:** Contains zinc, which helps keep the scalp healthy and supports hair growth.

How to Include:

- **Boiled or Scrambled:** Enjoy eggs boiled, scrambled, or poached for breakfast.
- **Omelets:** Make vegetable-packed omelets for a nutritious meal.
- **Baking:** Use eggs in baking recipes to ensure you're getting this vital nutrient.

3. Spinach

Nutrient Benefits:

- **Iron:** Spinach is rich in iron, which helps red blood cells carry oxygen to hair follicles, promoting growth.
- **Vitamin A:** Contains vitamin A, which helps in the production of sebum, keeping the scalp moisturized.
- **Vitamin C:** High in vitamin C, which aids in collagen production and strengthens hair.

How to Include:

- **Salads:** Add fresh spinach to salads for a nutrient boost.
- **Smoothies:** Blend spinach into smoothies for a healthy, green addition.
- **Cooked Dishes:** Incorporate spinach into soups, stews, and casseroles.

4. Sweet Potatoes

Nutrient Benefits:

- **Beta-Carotene:** Sweet potatoes are high in beta-carotene, which the body converts to vitamin A. This helps produce sebum, which keeps hair healthy.
- **Antioxidants:** The antioxidants in sweet potatoes help protect hair follicles from damage.

How to Include:

- **Baked:** Enjoy baked sweet potatoes as a side dish.
- **Mashed:** Make mashed sweet potatoes for a delicious and nutritious meal.
- **Fries:** Bake sweet potato fries for a healthy snack.

5. Avocados

Nutrient Benefits:

- **Healthy Fats:** Avocados are rich in healthy fats that moisturize the scalp and hair, promoting shine and elasticity.
- **Vitamin E:** Contains vitamin E, which improves blood circulation to the scalp and helps hair grow faster.
- **Biotin:** High in biotin, which strengthens hair and promotes growth.

How to Include:

- **Guacamole:** Make guacamole for a tasty dip or spread.
- **Salads:** Add sliced avocado to salads for a creamy texture.
- **Smoothies:** Blend avocado into smoothies for added creaminess and nutrition.

6. Nuts and Seeds

Nutrient Benefits:

- **Omega-3 Fatty Acids:** Nuts and seeds like walnuts and flaxseeds are high in omega-3 fatty acids, which support scalp health and hair growth.
- **Vitamin E:** Rich in vitamin E, which protects hair from oxidative stress.
- **Zinc:** Contains zinc, which helps keep hair healthy and promotes growth.

How to Include:

- **Snacking:** Enjoy a handful of nuts as a healthy snack.
- **Toppings:** Sprinkle seeds on top of salads, yogurt, or oatmeal.
- **Baking:** Incorporate nuts and seeds into baking recipes for added nutrition.

7. Greek Yogurt

Nutrient Benefits:

- **Protein:** Greek yogurt is high in protein, which is essential for hair strength and growth.
- **Vitamin B5:** Contains vitamin B5 (pantothenic acid), which helps improve blood flow to the scalp and promote hair growth.
- **Probiotics:** The probiotics in Greek yogurt help maintain a healthy scalp environment.

How to Include:

- **Breakfast:** Enjoy Greek yogurt with fruit and honey for breakfast.
- **Smoothies:** Blend Greek yogurt into smoothies for a creamy texture.
- **Snacks:** Use Greek yogurt as a base for dips and dressings.

8. Berries

Nutrient Benefits:

- **Vitamin C:** Berries like strawberries, blueberries, and raspberries are rich in vitamin C, which aids in collagen production and strengthens hair.
- **Antioxidants:** The antioxidants in berries help protect hair follicles from damage.

How to Include:

- **Fresh:** Eat berries fresh as a snack or dessert.
- **Smoothies:** Blend berries into smoothies for a nutrient-packed drink.
- **Toppings:** Add berries to yogurt, cereal, or oatmeal.

9. Lean Meats

Nutrient Benefits:

- **Protein:** Lean meats like chicken and turkey provide high-quality protein, which is essential for hair structure.
- **Iron:** Rich in iron, which helps transport oxygen to hair follicles, promoting growth.

How to Include:

- **Grilled or Baked:** Enjoy grilled or baked chicken or turkey as a main dish.
- **Salads:** Add cooked lean meats to salads for a protein boost.
- **Sandwiches:** Use lean meats in sandwiches for a nutritious meal.

10. Legumes

Nutrient Benefits:

- **Protein:** Legumes like lentils, beans, and chickpeas are excellent sources of plant-based protein, which supports hair growth.
- **Iron:** High in iron, which is necessary for healthy hair follicles.
- **Zinc:** Contains zinc, which helps keep the scalp healthy and supports hair growth.

How to Include:

- **Soups and Stews:** Add legumes to soups and stews for a hearty meal.
- **Salads:** Mix cooked legumes into salads for added texture and nutrition.
- **Dips:** Make hummus or other bean-based dips for a healthy snack.

Nutritional supplements

In addition to a balanced diet, certain nutritional supplements can provide additional support for hair growth and overall hair health. These supplements contain essential vitamins, minerals, and other compounds that are beneficial for maintaining strong, healthy hair. Here's a detailed guide on the best nutritional supplements to consider for promoting hair health.

1. Biotin (Vitamin B7)

Benefits:

- **Promotes Hair Growth:** Biotin is essential for the production of keratin, a protein that makes up hair. It helps stimulate hair growth and increases hair thickness.
- **Prevents Hair Loss:** Biotin deficiency can lead to hair thinning and loss. Supplementing with biotin can help prevent these issues.

Recommended Dosage:

- **Daily Intake:** The typical recommended dosage for biotin supplements is 2,500 to 5,000 mcg per day. Consult with a healthcare professional before starting any new supplement.

2. Vitamin D

Benefits:

- **Stimulates Hair Follicles:** Vitamin D helps create new hair follicles, which can improve hair thickness and prevent hair loss.
- **Reduces Hair Shedding:** Adequate levels of vitamin D can reduce hair shedding and promote healthy hair growth.

Recommended Dosage:

- **Daily Intake:** The recommended daily intake of vitamin D varies depending on age, sex, and individual needs but generally ranges from 600 to 2,000 IU. A healthcare provider can determine the appropriate dosage based on blood tests.

3. Omega-3 Fatty Acids

Benefits:

- **Nourishes Hair Follicles:** Omega-3 fatty acids found in fish oil supplements nourish hair follicles and promote healthy hair growth.
- **Reduces Inflammation:** These fatty acids have anti-inflammatory properties that can help reduce scalp inflammation and prevent hair loss.

Recommended Dosage:

- **Daily Intake:** The typical dosage for omega-3 supplements is 1,000 to 2,000 mg per day. Ensure the supplement contains both EPA and DHA for maximum benefit.

4. Iron

Benefits:

- **Improves Blood Flow:** Iron is crucial for red blood cell production, which improves blood flow to the scalp and hair follicles, promoting growth.
- **Prevents Hair Loss:** Iron deficiency is a common cause of hair loss, particularly in women. Supplementing with iron can help prevent this.

Recommended Dosage:

- **Daily Intake:** The recommended daily intake of iron varies but is generally 18 mg for women and 8 mg for men. It's important to get a blood test and consult with a healthcare provider before starting iron supplements.

5. Zinc

Benefits:

- **Supports Hair Growth:** Zinc plays a vital role in hair tissue growth and repair.
- **Maintains Oil Glands:** Helps maintain the oil glands around hair follicles, ensuring a healthy scalp environment.

Recommended Dosage:

- **Daily Intake:** The recommended daily intake of zinc is 8-11 mg for adults. Over-supplementation can lead to adverse effects, so consult with a healthcare provider before starting.

6. Vitamin E

Benefits:

- **Promotes Scalp Health:** Vitamin E supports a healthy scalp environment by reducing oxidative stress and maintaining the protective lipid layer.
- **Improves Hair Growth:** Acts as an antioxidant, protecting hair follicles from damage and promoting hair growth.

Recommended Dosage:

- **Daily Intake:** The typical dosage for vitamin E supplements is 15 mg (22.4 IU) per day. Ensure to choose a natural form of vitamin E (d-alpha-tocopherol) for better absorption.

7. Collagen

Benefits:

- **Strengthens Hair:** Collagen is a major component of hair structure and helps strengthen hair, reducing breakage.
- **Promotes Growth:** Provides amino acids that are essential for building hair proteins.

Recommended Dosage:

- **Daily Intake:** The typical dosage for collagen supplements is 2.5 to 15 grams per day. Collagen peptides in powder form can be added to smoothies, coffee, or other beverages.

8. Folic Acid (Vitamin B9)

Benefits:

- **Promotes Cell Growth:** Folic acid plays a crucial role in cell growth, which is essential for healthy hair growth.

- **Prevents Hair Thinning:** Helps prevent hair thinning by supporting the health of hair follicles.

Recommended Dosage:

- **Daily Intake:** The recommended daily intake for folic acid is 400 mcg for adults. It's often included in multivitamins and prenatal vitamins.

9. Vitamin C

Benefits:

- **Enhances Iron Absorption:** Vitamin C helps the body absorb iron more efficiently, which is essential for hair growth.
- **Promotes Collagen Production:** Essential for collagen production, which strengthens hair and promotes growth.

Recommended Dosage:

- **Daily Intake:** The recommended daily intake of vitamin C is 75 mg for women and 90 mg for men. Vitamin C supplements are available in various forms, including tablets and gummies.

10. Keratin Supplements

Benefits:

- **Strengthens Hair:** Keratin is the primary protein that makes up hair, and supplementing with keratin can help strengthen hair strands.
- **Reduces Breakage:** Helps reduce hair breakage and improves overall hair texture and shine.

Recommended Dosage:

- **Daily Intake:** The typical dosage for keratin supplements varies, but 500 to 1,000 mg per day is common. Always follow the manufacturer's recommendations and consult with a healthcare provider.

Stress Management

Impact of stress on hair growth

Stress is a common part of life, but chronic stress can have a significant impact on hair growth and overall hair health. Understanding the connection between stress and hair loss, and adopting effective stress management techniques, can help maintain healthy hair. Here's a detailed guide on how stress affects hair growth and strategies to manage stress.

1. How Stress Affects Hair Growth

Hormonal Imbalance:

- **Cortisol Production:** When you experience stress, your body produces higher levels of cortisol, the stress hormone. Elevated cortisol levels can disrupt the hair growth cycle, leading to hair loss.
- **Hormonal Disruption:** Stress can also affect the balance of other hormones, such as androgens, which can contribute to hair thinning and loss.

Hair Growth Cycle Disruption:

- **Telogen Effluvium:** Chronic stress can push a large number of hair follicles into the telogen (resting) phase prematurely, leading to increased hair shedding, known as telogen effluvium.
- **Anagen Effluvium:** In some cases, severe stress can disrupt the anagen (growth) phase, causing hair to stop growing and fall out.

Nutrient Depletion:

- **Poor Absorption:** Stress can affect the digestive system, leading to poor nutrient absorption. This can result in deficiencies of essential vitamins and minerals needed for healthy hair growth.
- **Weakened Immune System:** Chronic stress weakens the immune system, making the scalp more susceptible to infections and conditions like dandruff and seborrheic dermatitis, which can impact hair growth.

2. Stress Management Techniques

Regular Exercise:

- **Physical Activity:** Engaging in regular physical activity, such as walking, jogging, yoga, or strength training, helps reduce stress levels by releasing endorphins, the body's natural stress relievers.
- **Mind-Body Exercises:** Practices like yoga, tai chi, and pilates combine physical movement with mindfulness and deep breathing, promoting relaxation and reducing stress.

Healthy Diet:

- **Balanced Nutrition:** Eating a balanced diet rich in fruits, vegetables, whole grains, lean proteins, and healthy fats provides the necessary nutrients to support hair health and reduce the effects of stress.
- **Hydration:** Staying well-hydrated helps maintain overall health and supports the body's stress response.

Mindfulness and Relaxation Techniques:

- **Meditation:** Regular meditation practice can help calm the mind, reduce stress, and improve overall well-being. Even a few minutes a day can make a significant difference.
- **Deep Breathing:** Techniques such as diaphragmatic breathing or the 4-7-8 breathing method can help activate the body's relaxation response and reduce stress.

Adequate Sleep:

- **Sleep Quality:** Ensuring you get 7-9 hours of quality sleep each night is crucial for stress management. Poor sleep can exacerbate stress levels and impact hair health.
- **Sleep Hygiene:** Create a relaxing bedtime routine, avoid screens before bed, and maintain a consistent sleep schedule to improve sleep quality.

Professional Support:

- **Therapy and Counseling:** Speaking with a mental health professional can help you develop coping strategies for managing stress and addressing underlying issues.
- **Support Groups:** Joining support groups or communities can provide a sense of connection and reduce feelings of isolation and stress.

Hobbies and Leisure Activities:

- **Engage in Enjoyable Activities:** Spending time on hobbies and activities you enjoy can provide a mental break from stressors and improve your overall mood.
- **Creative Outlets:** Activities such as painting, writing, playing music, or gardening can be therapeutic and reduce stress levels.

Time Management:

- **Prioritization:** Organize your tasks and responsibilities to avoid feeling overwhelmed. Prioritize important tasks and delegate when possible.
- **Breaks and Downtime:** Incorporate regular breaks and downtime into your schedule to relax and recharge.

Social Connections:

- **Stay Connected:** Maintain strong social connections with friends and family. Social support can buffer against stress and provide emotional support.
- **Talk About It:** Sharing your feelings and concerns with someone you trust can alleviate stress and provide new perspectives.

Stress reduction techniques

Effectively managing and reducing stress is crucial for maintaining overall health and promoting healthy hair growth. Here are several stress reduction techniques that can help you manage stress levels, enhance your well-being, and support hair health.

1. Regular Exercise

Benefits:

- **Endorphin Release:** Physical activity releases endorphins, the body's natural stress relievers, which can improve mood and reduce stress.
- **Improved Sleep:** Exercise can help regulate sleep patterns, leading to better quality sleep, which is essential for stress management.

Techniques:

- **Cardio Workouts:** Engage in cardiovascular exercises such as running, cycling, or swimming for at least 30 minutes, 3-5 times a week.
- **Strength Training:** Incorporate strength training exercises such as weightlifting or bodyweight exercises to build muscle and improve overall fitness.
- **Mind-Body Exercises:** Practice yoga, pilates, or tai chi to combine physical activity with mindfulness and relaxation.

2. Healthy Diet

Benefits:

- **Balanced Nutrition:** A diet rich in fruits, vegetables, whole grains, lean proteins, and healthy fats provides the necessary nutrients to support stress management and overall health.
- **Energy and Mood Regulation:** Proper nutrition helps regulate energy levels and mood, reducing the impact of stress.

Techniques:

- **Eat Regular Meals:** Ensure you eat regular, balanced meals throughout the day to maintain stable blood sugar levels and energy.
- **Stay Hydrated:** Drink plenty of water to stay hydrated, which is essential for physical and mental health.
- **Limit Caffeine and Sugar:** Reduce intake of caffeine and sugary foods, which can contribute to stress and anxiety.

3. Mindfulness and Relaxation Techniques

Benefits:

- **Calm the Mind:** Mindfulness and relaxation practices can help calm the mind, reduce stress, and improve overall well-being.

- **Focus on the Present:** These techniques encourage focusing on the present moment, reducing anxiety about the past or future.

Techniques:

- **Meditation:** Practice meditation daily, starting with just a few minutes and gradually increasing the duration. Use guided meditation apps or videos if needed.
- **Deep Breathing:** Practice deep breathing exercises such as diaphragmatic breathing or the 4-7-8 breathing technique to activate the body's relaxation response.
- **Progressive Muscle Relaxation:** Sequentially tense and then relax each muscle group in your body to reduce physical tension and stress.

4. Adequate Sleep

Benefits:

- **Rest and Recovery:** Quality sleep is essential for the body and mind to rest and recover, reducing stress levels.
- **Improved Mood:** Adequate sleep helps regulate mood and improves emotional resilience.

Techniques:

- **Sleep Routine:** Establish a regular sleep routine by going to bed and waking up at the same time every day, even on weekends.
- **Sleep Environment:** Create a relaxing sleep environment by keeping the bedroom cool, dark, and quiet. Use comfortable bedding and limit screen time before bed.
- **Relaxation Techniques:** Practice relaxation techniques such as reading, listening to calming music, or taking a warm bath before bedtime.

5. Professional Support

Benefits:

- **Guidance and Strategies:** Professional support from therapists or counselors can provide guidance and strategies for managing stress.
- **Emotional Support:** Talking to a professional can help you process emotions and reduce feelings of isolation.

Techniques:

- **Therapy:** Seek individual therapy or counseling to address specific stressors and develop coping strategies.
- **Support Groups:** Join support groups or community groups to connect with others who are experiencing similar challenges and gain emotional support.
- **Online Resources:** Utilize online therapy platforms or hotlines if in-person therapy is not accessible.

6. Hobbies and Leisure Activities

Benefits:

- **Mental Break:** Engaging in enjoyable activities provides a mental break from stressors and improves overall mood.
- **Creative Expression:** Hobbies can offer an outlet for creative expression and relaxation.

Techniques:

- **Find a Hobby:** Explore different hobbies such as painting, writing, gardening, cooking, or playing a musical instrument to find what you enjoy.
- **Schedule Time:** Dedicate regular time each week to engage in your chosen hobbies and leisure activities.
- **Join a Group:** Consider joining a club or group related to your hobby to meet like-minded individuals and expand your social network.

7. Time Management

Benefits:

- **Reduced Overwhelm:** Effective time management helps reduce feelings of overwhelm and stress by organizing tasks and responsibilities.
- **Increased Productivity:** Prioritizing tasks and managing time effectively can increase productivity and create a sense of accomplishment.

Techniques:

- **Prioritize Tasks:** Make a list of tasks and prioritize them based on importance and deadlines. Focus on completing high-priority tasks first.
- **Break Tasks Down:** Break larger tasks into smaller, manageable steps to make them less daunting.
- **Set Boundaries:** Learn to say no to additional commitments that may add to your stress levels and ensure you have time for self-care.

8. Social Connections

Benefits:

- **Emotional Support:** Strong social connections provide emotional support, reducing feelings of isolation and stress.
- **Shared Experiences:** Sharing experiences and feelings with friends and family can provide new perspectives and coping strategies.

Techniques:

- **Stay Connected:** Regularly connect with friends and family through phone calls, video chats, or in-person visits.

- **Join Social Groups:** Participate in social groups, clubs, or community activities to meet new people and expand your support network.
- **Communicate Openly:** Share your feelings and concerns with trusted individuals to gain support and reduce stress.

Conclusion

Effectively managing and reducing stress is essential for maintaining overall health and promoting healthy hair growth. Techniques such as regular exercise, a healthy diet, mindfulness and relaxation practices, adequate sleep, professional support, engaging in hobbies, time management, and maintaining social connections can help you manage stress levels and enhance your well-being. Incorporating these practices into your daily routine can lead to significant improvements in both your mental health and hair health.

Regular Hair Care Routine

Daily and weekly hair care tips

Maintaining a regular hair care routine is essential for promoting healthy hair growth and keeping your hair in its best condition. A consistent routine helps prevent damage, nourishes the hair and scalp, and supports overall hair health. Here's a detailed guide on daily and weekly hair care tips to incorporate into your routine.

1. Daily Hair Care Tips

Gentle Cleansing:

- **Choose the Right Shampoo:** Use a gentle, sulfate-free shampoo that suits your hair type and addresses any specific concerns (e.g., dryness, dandruff, color-treated hair).
- **Avoid Over-Washing:** Wash your hair only as needed to avoid stripping it of its natural oils. For most people, washing 2-3 times a week is sufficient.

Conditioning:

- **Regular Conditioner:** Apply a moisturizing conditioner after every shampoo to keep your hair hydrated and manageable. Focus on the mid-lengths to ends, avoiding the scalp.
- **Leave-In Conditioner:** Use a leave-in conditioner or detangling spray on damp hair to provide extra moisture and make detangling easier.

Scalp Care:

- **Scalp Massage:** Gently massage your scalp for a few minutes daily to stimulate blood flow and promote healthy hair growth. Use your fingertips in circular motions.

Detangling:

- **Wide-Tooth Comb:** Use a wide-tooth comb to detangle wet hair, starting from the ends and working your way up to prevent breakage.
- **Avoid Rough Toweling:** Pat your hair dry with a microfiber towel or a soft cotton T-shirt instead of rubbing it with a regular towel.

Heat Protection:

- **Heat Protectant:** Apply a heat protectant spray or serum before using heat styling tools like blow dryers, straighteners, or curling irons to minimize damage.
- **Limit Heat Styling:** Try to minimize the use of heat styling tools. Opt for air-drying or heatless styling methods whenever possible.

Hair Oils and Serums:

- **Hydrating Oils:** Apply a small amount of hydrating oil, such as argan oil or castor oil, to the ends of your hair to keep them moisturized and prevent split ends.
- **Serums:** Use a lightweight serum to add shine and smoothness to your hair, focusing on the ends and any frizzy areas.

2. Weekly Hair Care Tips

Deep Conditioning:

- **Deep Conditioning Treatment:** Apply a deep conditioning mask or treatment once a week to provide intense hydration and repair. Leave it on for the recommended time before rinsing thoroughly.
- **Castor Oil Treatment:** Use a castor oil treatment weekly. Apply castor oil to your scalp and hair, cover with a shower cap, and leave it on for at least 30 minutes or overnight before washing.

Exfoliating the Scalp:

- **Scalp Scrub:** Use a gentle scalp scrub or exfoliating treatment once a week to remove product buildup and dead skin cells. Massage the scrub into your scalp, then rinse thoroughly.

Clarifying Shampoo:

- **Monthly Clarifying:** Use a clarifying shampoo once a month to remove buildup from hair products, hard water minerals, and pollutants. Follow with a deep conditioner to restore moisture.

Protective Styles:

- **Low Manipulation Styles:** Opt for low manipulation styles like braids, twists, or buns to protect your hair from breakage and reduce daily styling stress.
- **Night Protection:** Use a silk or satin pillowcase, or wear a silk or satin scarf or bonnet while sleeping to reduce friction and prevent breakage.

Trimming:

- **Regular Trims:** Schedule regular trims every 6-8 weeks to remove split ends and maintain healthy hair. Trimming prevents split ends from traveling up the hair shaft, reducing overall damage.

Hydration and Diet:

- **Stay Hydrated:** Drink plenty of water daily to keep your hair and scalp hydrated from within.
- **Healthy Diet:** Eat a balanced diet rich in vitamins and minerals that support hair health, including biotin, vitamin D, omega-3 fatty acids, and iron.

Avoiding Harsh Chemicals:

- **Limit Chemical Treatments:** Minimize the use of harsh chemical treatments such as coloring, perming, or relaxing. If you do use these treatments, ensure proper aftercare and conditioning.
- **Natural Alternatives:** Opt for natural hair care products and treatments whenever possible to reduce exposure to harsh chemicals.

Stress Management:

- **Manage Stress:** Incorporate stress management techniques such as exercise, meditation, and hobbies to reduce stress levels, which can impact hair health.

Maintenance for long-term health

Maintaining long-term hair health requires consistent care, attention to detail, and adopting healthy habits that support the overall well-being of your hair and scalp. Here's an in-depth guide on how to maintain your hair's health over the long term, ensuring it stays strong, vibrant, and resilient.

1. Consistent Hair Care Routine

Daily Care:

- **Gentle Shampooing:** Continue using a gentle, sulfate-free shampoo that suits your hair type. Avoid over-washing to prevent stripping natural oils.
- **Conditioning:** Always condition your hair after shampooing to keep it hydrated and manageable. Use a leave-in conditioner for added moisture and protection.

Weekly Treatments:

- **Deep Conditioning:** Apply a deep conditioning mask or treatment weekly to provide intense hydration and repair. Use castor oil treatments regularly to strengthen and nourish your hair.

- **Scalp Care:** Exfoliate your scalp weekly with a gentle scrub to remove buildup and promote a healthy environment for hair growth.

2. Regular Trims

Prevent Split Ends:

- **Scheduled Trims:** Trim your hair every 6-8 weeks to remove split ends and prevent them from traveling up the hair shaft. Regular trims keep your hair looking healthy and reduce breakage.

Professional Cuts:

- **Visit a Stylist:** Regular visits to a professional stylist can ensure your hair is trimmed properly and any specific hair concerns are addressed.

3. Balanced Diet and Supplements

Nutrient-Rich Foods:

- **Healthy Eating:** Maintain a balanced diet rich in vitamins and minerals essential for hair health. Include foods high in biotin, vitamin D, omega-3 fatty acids, iron, zinc, and protein.
- **Hydration:** Drink plenty of water daily to keep your hair and scalp hydrated from within.

Supplements:

- **Targeted Supplements:** Consider taking nutritional supplements like biotin, vitamin D, omega-3 fatty acids, and collagen to support hair growth and health. Consult with a healthcare professional before starting any new supplement regimen.

4. Protecting Hair from Damage

Heat Protection:

- **Limit Heat Styling:** Minimize the use of heat styling tools like blow dryers, straighteners, and curling irons. When you do use them, always apply a heat protectant spray to minimize damage.
- **Air-Drying:** Opt for air-drying your hair whenever possible to reduce heat exposure.

Chemical Treatments:

- **Reduce Chemical Use:** Limit the use of chemical treatments such as coloring, perming, or relaxing. If you use these treatments, ensure proper aftercare with deep conditioning and hydration.
- **Natural Alternatives:** Choose natural hair care products and treatments to avoid exposure to harsh chemicals.

5. Gentle Handling of Hair

Detangling:

- **Wide-Tooth Comb:** Use a wide-tooth comb to detangle wet hair, starting from the ends and working your way up to prevent breakage.
- **Soft Toweling:** Gently pat your hair dry with a microfiber towel or a soft cotton T-shirt instead of rubbing it with a regular towel.

Styling:

- **Protective Styles:** Opt for low manipulation and protective styles such as braids, twists, or buns to minimize breakage and reduce daily styling stress.
- **Night Protection:** Use a silk or satin pillowcase, or wear a silk or satin scarf or bonnet while sleeping to reduce friction and prevent breakage.

6. Scalp Health

Regular Scalp Massage:

- **Stimulate Growth:** Massage your scalp regularly to stimulate blood flow, promote healthy hair growth, and reduce tension. Use your fingertips in circular motions for a few minutes daily.

Scalp Treatments:

- **Targeted Treatments:** Use scalp treatments and serums designed to address specific scalp issues like dryness, dandruff, or sensitivity. Look for products with soothing and hydrating ingredients.

7. Stress Management

Reduce Stress:

- **Mindfulness Practices:** Incorporate mindfulness practices such as meditation, deep breathing exercises, and yoga to manage stress effectively.
- **Hobbies and Leisure:** Engage in hobbies and leisure activities that you enjoy to provide a mental break from stressors.

Professional Support:

- **Therapy and Counseling:** Seek professional support if you experience chronic stress or emotional challenges. Therapists and counselors can help you develop coping strategies.

8. Environmental Protection

Protect from Sun Exposure:

- **UV Protection:** Protect your hair from UV damage by wearing a hat or using hair products with UV filters when spending extended time outdoors.

Shield from Pollution:

- **Anti-Pollution Products:** Use hair care products designed to shield hair from environmental pollutants. Rinse your hair thoroughly after exposure to pollution to remove residue.

Conclusion

Recap and Final Thoughts

Summary of key points

The journey to healthier, stronger, and more vibrant hair involves understanding and applying various techniques and practices. From the benefits of castor oil to daily hair care routines, dietary considerations, and stress management, each aspect plays a crucial role in promoting hair growth and maintaining overall hair health. Here's a summary of the key points discussed throughout this book:

1. The Science of Hair Growth

- **Hair Structure and Composition:** Understanding the anatomy of hair, including the cuticle, cortex, and medulla, helps in choosing appropriate hair care practices.
- **Hair Growth Cycle:** Recognizing the stages of hair growth—anagen, catagen, and telogen—enables better management of hair growth and shedding.

2. Common Hair Problems

- **Hair Loss:** Identifying types of hair loss (e.g., androgenetic alopecia, telogen effluvium) and their causes is essential for effective treatment.
- **Thinning Hair:** Understanding the reasons behind thinning hair and exploring treatment options, such as topical treatments and lifestyle changes.
- **Damaged Hair:** Learning about causes of hair damage, including heat, chemicals, and environmental factors, and strategies for repair and prevention.

3. Natural Hair Care Basics

- **Benefits of Natural Hair Care:** Emphasizing the advantages of using natural products over synthetic ones, including reduced chemical exposure and long-term hair health.
- **Key Natural Ingredients:** Exploring beneficial natural ingredients like aloe vera, coconut oil, and honey, and their specific benefits for hair health.

4. Castor Oil Fundamentals

- **What is Castor Oil?:** Understanding the history, origins, and types of castor oil, such as cold-pressed and refined, and their chemical composition.
- **Benefits of Castor Oil for Hair:** Highlighting castor oil's ability to promote hair growth, strengthen hair, moisturize and condition, and treat scalp conditions.

5. Practical Applications of Castor Oil

- **Preparation and Application Techniques:** Detailed methods for preparing and applying castor oil, including frequency and dosage recommendations.

- **Castor Oil Hair Treatments:** Techniques like scalp massages, overnight treatments, and hot oil treatments to maximize the benefits of castor oil.
- **DIY Castor Oil Hair Recipes:** Creating effective hair masks, conditioners, serums, and sprays using castor oil and other natural ingredients.

6. Enhancing the Effects of Castor Oil

- **Combining with Other Ingredients:** Using essential oils, carrier oils, and herbal infusions to enhance the benefits of castor oil.
- **Healthy Lifestyle Practices:** Incorporating a balanced diet, nutritional supplements, stress management techniques, and regular hair care routines to support hair health.

7. Regular Hair Care Routine

- **Daily Hair Care Tips:** Gentle cleansing, conditioning, scalp care, detangling, and heat protection for everyday maintenance.
- **Weekly Hair Care Tips:** Deep conditioning, scalp exfoliation, protective styles, and regular trims for ongoing hair health.

8. Long-Term Hair Health Maintenance

- **Consistent Routine:** Maintaining a consistent hair care routine that includes regular treatments and protection from damage.
- **Balanced Diet and Supplements:** Ensuring a nutrient-rich diet and considering supplements to support hair health.
- **Gentle Handling and Environmental Protection:** Gentle hair handling techniques and protecting hair from environmental damage and harsh chemicals.

Final Thoughts

Healthy hair is a reflection of overall well-being and requires a holistic approach that includes proper care, nutrition, and stress management. By understanding the science behind hair growth and the benefits of natural ingredients like castor oil, you can develop a comprehensive hair care routine that supports long-term hair health.

Remember, consistency is key. Regularly incorporating these practices into your daily and weekly routines will yield the best results over time. Whether you are dealing with specific hair issues or simply want to maintain the health and vitality of your hair, the knowledge and techniques shared in this book provide a solid foundation for achieving your hair goals.

Key Takeaways

Throughout this book, we have explored the numerous benefits of castor oil for hair growth, the science behind hair health, and the importance of a comprehensive hair care routine. Here are the key takeaways from the Castor Oil for Hair Growth Bible, summarizing the main messages and essential insights for maintaining healthy, vibrant hair.

1. Understanding Hair and Hair Growth

Hair Structure and Composition:

- Hair is composed of the cuticle, cortex, and medulla. Each part plays a crucial role in the hair's overall health and appearance.

Hair Growth Cycle:

- The hair growth cycle consists of three stages: anagen (growth), catagen (transition), and telogen (resting). Understanding this cycle helps in managing hair growth and addressing hair loss.

Factors Affecting Hair Growth:

- Both internal factors (hormones, genetics, nutrition) and external factors (environment, hair care practices) influence hair growth. Maintaining a balanced lifestyle and proper hair care can optimize hair health.

Common Hair Problems:

- Hair loss, thinning hair, and damaged hair are common issues that can be managed with appropriate treatments and lifestyle changes.

2. Benefits of Natural Hair Care

Natural Ingredients:

- Using natural ingredients like aloe vera, coconut oil, and honey can provide gentle and effective care for your hair, reducing exposure to harsh chemicals.

Why Choose Castor Oil?:

- Castor oil is a powerful natural remedy known for its ability to promote hair growth, strengthen hair, moisturize, condition, and treat scalp conditions.

3. Castor Oil Fundamentals

What is Castor Oil?:

- Castor oil, derived from the castor bean plant, comes in various forms such as cold-pressed and refined. Its chemical composition includes ricinoleic acid, which provides numerous benefits for hair health.

Benefits of Castor Oil:

- Castor oil promotes hair growth, strengthens hair, moisturizes and conditions, and treats scalp conditions like dandruff and itchiness.

4. Practical Applications of Castor Oil

Preparation and Application Techniques:

- Proper preparation and application techniques ensure that castor oil is used effectively. Techniques include scalp massages, overnight treatments, and hot oil treatments.

DIY Castor Oil Hair Recipes:

- Homemade hair masks, conditioners, serums, and sprays using castor oil can address specific hair concerns and provide tailored benefits.

5. Enhancing the Effects of Castor Oil

Combining with Other Ingredients:

- Essential oils, carrier oils, and herbal infusions can enhance the benefits of castor oil, providing additional nourishment and addressing specific hair concerns.

Healthy Lifestyle Practices:

- A balanced diet, nutritional supplements, stress management, and regular hair care routines are essential for supporting hair health and maximizing the benefits of castor oil.

6. Regular Hair Care Routine

Daily Hair Care Tips:

- Gentle cleansing, regular conditioning, scalp care, proper detangling, and heat protection are vital for maintaining healthy hair.

Weekly Hair Care Tips:

- Deep conditioning treatments, scalp exfoliation, protective styles, and regular trims contribute to ongoing hair health.

7. Maintenance for Long-Term Health

Consistent Routine:

- Maintaining a consistent hair care routine with regular treatments and protection from damage ensures long-term hair health.

Balanced Diet and Supplements:

- Nutrient-rich foods and targeted supplements support hair health from within, promoting growth and strength.

Gentle Handling and Environmental Protection:

- Gentle handling techniques and protection from environmental damage and harsh chemicals are crucial for maintaining hair health.

Additional Resources

1. Appendices
   - FAQs
     - Common Questions and Answers about Castor Oil and Hair Growth

1. What is castor oil, and how does it benefit hair growth?

Answer: Castor oil is a natural oil extracted from the seeds of the castor bean plant (Ricinus communis). It is rich in ricinoleic acid, a type of fatty acid that provides several benefits for hair growth and health:

- **Promotes Hair Growth:** Ricinoleic acid increases blood circulation to the scalp, which stimulates hair follicles and promotes growth.
- **Moisturizes and Conditions:** Castor oil is a natural humectant, drawing moisture into the hair and keeping it hydrated, soft, and manageable.
- **Strengthens Hair:** The fatty acids in castor oil help strengthen hair strands, reducing breakage and split ends.
- **Treats Scalp Conditions:** Its anti-inflammatory and antimicrobial properties help treat scalp conditions like dandruff and itchiness.

2. How should I apply castor oil to my hair and scalp?

Answer: Applying castor oil effectively involves a few steps:

- **Preparation:** Warm the castor oil slightly to enhance absorption.
- **Application:** Part your hair into sections and apply the oil directly to your scalp using an applicator bottle or your fingertips. Massage the oil into your scalp in circular motions to stimulate blood flow.

- **Distribution:** Apply the oil to the lengths and ends of your hair to ensure even coverage.
- **Leave-On Time:** Leave the oil on for at least 30 minutes, or overnight for a deep conditioning treatment.
- **Rinse:** Wash your hair thoroughly with a gentle shampoo to remove the oil.

3. How often should I use castor oil on my hair?

Answer: The frequency of castor oil application depends on your hair type and needs:

- **For Hair Growth:** Apply castor oil 2-3 times a week to stimulate hair growth and improve scalp health.
- **For Moisturizing and Conditioning:** Use castor oil as a weekly deep conditioning treatment.
- **For Treating Scalp Conditions:** Apply castor oil once a week to maintain scalp health and treat conditions like dandruff.

4. Can castor oil be mixed with other oils or ingredients?

Answer: Yes, castor oil can be mixed with other oils and natural ingredients to enhance its benefits:

- **Carrier Oils:** Mix castor oil with carrier oils like coconut oil, jojoba oil, or argan oil to improve its consistency and add additional nutrients.
- **Essential Oils:** Add essential oils like rosemary, lavender, or peppermint to enhance hair growth, soothe the scalp, and add fragrance.
- **Herbal Infusions:** Combine castor oil with herbal infusions made from herbs like rosemary, chamomile, or nettle to provide additional benefits for hair health.

5. Are there any side effects of using castor oil on hair?

Answer: Castor oil is generally safe for most people, but some may experience side effects:

- **Allergic Reactions:** A small number of people may be allergic to castor oil. Conduct a patch test before using it on your scalp or hair.
- **Scalp Irritation:** Overuse or improper application can cause scalp irritation. Use the oil in moderation and ensure thorough rinsing.
- **Greasy Residue:** Castor oil is thick and can leave a greasy residue if not rinsed out properly. Use a clarifying shampoo to ensure complete removal.

6. Can castor oil help with hair thinning and bald spots?

Answer: Castor oil can be effective in promoting hair growth and reducing thinning:

- **Stimulation of Hair Follicles:** Massaging castor oil into the scalp can stimulate hair follicles and promote the growth of new hair.
- **Nourishment:** The nutrients in castor oil strengthen existing hair, reduce breakage, and improve overall hair density.

- **Consistency:** Regular use is key. Apply castor oil 2-3 times a week and be patient, as hair growth takes time.

7. Is castor oil suitable for all hair types?

Answer: Yes, castor oil is suitable for all hair types, but its use may vary:

- **Dry Hair:** Castor oil is especially beneficial for dry, brittle hair due to its moisturizing properties.
- **Oily Hair:** Those with oily hair may need to use castor oil sparingly and focus on scalp treatments rather than applying it to the lengths of the hair.
- **Curly Hair:** Castor oil can help define curls and reduce frizz in curly hair types.

8. How does castor oil compare to other natural oils for hair care?

Answer: Castor oil has unique properties that make it stand out among other natural oils:

- **Thicker Consistency:** Castor oil is thicker than many other oils, making it excellent for deep conditioning and scalp treatments.
- **Higher Ricinoleic Acid Content:** The high content of ricinoleic acid in castor oil provides unique benefits for hair growth and scalp health.
- **Moisturizing and Protective:** While other oils like coconut oil and argan oil are also moisturizing, castor oil's thick consistency offers a protective barrier, sealing in moisture.

9. Can castor oil be used on colored or chemically treated hair?

Answer: Yes, castor oil can be beneficial for colored or chemically treated hair:

- **Moisturizing:** It helps restore moisture lost during chemical treatments.
- **Strengthening:** Castor oil strengthens weakened hair strands, reducing breakage and split ends.
- **Protection:** Its protective properties help shield hair from further damage.

10. How long does it take to see results with castor oil?

Answer: The time it takes to see results can vary based on individual factors:

- **Consistency:** Regular use is crucial. Apply castor oil 2-3 times a week.
- **Hair Growth Cycle:** Hair growth cycles vary, but you may start noticing improvements in hair texture and strength within a few weeks. Visible growth may take a few months.
- **Overall Health:** Factors such as diet, stress levels, and overall health can impact the effectiveness of castor oil treatments.

Glossary

Terms and Definitions

Understanding the terminology related to hair care and castor oil is essential for effectively using the information provided in this book. Here's a glossary of key terms and their definitions to help you navigate the concepts discussed.

1. Anagen Phase

Definition:

- The active growth phase of the hair cycle, during which the hair follicle is producing new hair. This phase can last several years and determines the length of the hair.

2. Antioxidants

Definition:

- Compounds that protect cells from damage caused by free radicals. Antioxidants are important for maintaining healthy hair and preventing damage.

3. Biotin

Definition:

- Also known as vitamin B7, biotin is a water-soluble vitamin that supports the production of keratin, a protein essential for hair growth and strength.

4. Carrier Oils

Definition:

- Base oils used to dilute essential oils and make them safe for topical application. Common carrier oils include coconut oil, jojoba oil, and argan oil.

5. Catagen Phase

Definition:

- The transitional phase of the hair growth cycle, lasting a few weeks. During this phase, hair growth stops, and the hair follicle begins to shrink.

6. Cold-Pressed

Definition:

- A method of extracting oil from seeds or nuts without using heat, preserving the oil's natural nutrients and beneficial properties.

7. Cortisol

Definition:

- A hormone produced by the adrenal glands in response to stress. High levels of cortisol can disrupt hair growth and contribute to hair loss.

8. Deep Conditioning

Definition:

- A hair treatment that provides intensive moisture and repair to the hair, typically applied once a week to restore and strengthen hair.

9. DHT (Dihydrotestosterone)

Definition:

- A hormone derived from testosterone that is linked to hair loss, particularly in cases of androgenetic alopecia (male and female pattern baldness).

10. Essential Oils

Definition:

- Concentrated plant extracts known for their aromatic properties and therapeutic benefits. Essential oils like rosemary, lavender, and peppermint can promote hair growth and scalp health.

11. Exfoliation

Definition:

- The process of removing dead skin cells from the scalp to improve scalp health and promote hair growth. Scalp exfoliation can be done using scrubs or specialized treatments.

12. Free Radicals

Definition:

- Unstable molecules that can damage cells, leading to aging and various health issues, including hair damage. Antioxidants help neutralize free radicals.

13. Humectant

Definition:

- A substance that attracts moisture from the air and binds it to the hair or skin. Castor oil is a natural humectant, helping to keep hair hydrated.

14. Keratin

Definition:

- A fibrous protein that forms the structure of hair, nails, and the outer layer of skin. Keratin strengthens hair and helps maintain its integrity.

15. Medulla

Definition:

- The innermost layer of the hair shaft, consisting of soft, spongy tissue. Not all hair types have a medulla.

16. Omega-3 Fatty Acids

Definition:

- Essential fats found in foods like fish and flaxseed. Omega-3 fatty acids nourish the hair follicles and promote healthy hair growth.

17. Patch Test

Definition:

- A method of testing a product on a small area of skin to check for allergic reactions before applying it more broadly.

18. Ricinoleic Acid

Definition:

- A fatty acid found in castor oil known for its anti-inflammatory and antimicrobial properties, as well as its ability to promote hair growth.

19. Sebum

Definition:

- The natural oil produced by the sebaceous glands in the scalp. Sebum helps keep the scalp and hair moisturized and protected.

20. Split Ends

Definition:

- The fraying or splitting of the hair shaft, typically at the ends, due to damage or dryness. Regular trims help prevent and manage split ends.

21. Telogen Phase

Definition:

- The resting phase of the hair growth cycle, during which the hair follicle is inactive. This phase lasts several months before the hair falls out and a new hair begins to grow.

22. Trichologist

Definition:

- A specialist in the study of hair and scalp health, providing diagnosis and treatment for hair and scalp disorders.

23. UV Protection

Definition:

- Protection from ultraviolet (UV) rays, which can damage hair and skin. Hair products with UV filters help shield hair from sun damage.

24. Wide-Tooth Comb

Definition:

- A comb with widely spaced teeth, used to detangle hair gently and minimize breakage, especially when hair is wet.

25. Zinc

Definition:

- A mineral essential for hair growth and repair. Zinc helps maintain the oil glands around hair follicles and supports overall hair health.